PRAISE FOR

The Pantry Principle

"Do you want to regain your health, or kickstart the journey to optimal health? Do you want to avoid eating foods containing Genetically Modified Organisms, toxins, heavy metals, artificial sweeteners or trans-fats? Mira has outlined an easy way to navigate those tricky food labels and to clean out your pantry of deleterious so-called foods. Mira not only gives you invaluable tips, but shares her story, which is one told all too many times today by individuals eating the Western Diet. I highly recommend you add this book to your health library."

— Gary Collins, M.S., Owner of New American Nutrition, author of *Factor X: The Last Health Program You Will Ever Need*

"This book is an excellent reference for anyone who shops, cooks and eats and wants to improve or maintain their health. I loved the up to date and practical information, written in simple to understand language, yet extensively referenced. The action plans at the end of each chapter are super. There is even information on how to save money and help the environment. Mira did her homework so the reader won't have to. Well done."

— Laura J. Knoff, B.Sc., Nutrition Consultant, author of *The Whole-Food Guide to Overcoming Irritable Bowel Syndrome: Strategies & Recipes for Eating Well With IBS, Indigestion & other Digestive Disorders*

"*The Pantry Principle* is a holistic home economics bible. If you are what you eat, and you eat from the 'poison pantry' described in the first part of this book, it's no surprise that discomfort, disorientation, and disease follow. By accepting Mira Dessy's invitation to a 'pantry party' you will learn to choose foods wisely, read labels, stock your refrigerator and shelves with fresh, whole, healing foods. Learn to protect or restore your family's health, as you follow the action plans to shop, cook, eat, and store a wide variety of unprocessed foods. By taking back control of your pantry, you are building a sustainable food source for your home, family, and friends. I look forward to recommending *The Pantry Principle* to my clients and students. Thanks for including a wide selection of references, resources, and fabulous recipes."

— Dr. Ed Bauman, Founder and President of Bauman College: Holistic Nutrition and Culinary Arts

"*The Pantry Principle* takes the confusion out of shopping...and eating. It demystifies the misleading and confusing labels and marketing lingo of the food industry, and helps families learn how to eat healthier. *The Pantry Principle* provides facts, better alternatives, and action steps to help you transform your diet and your life. I'd recommend it to any client that wants to help their family be healthier and happier."

— Julie Matthews, Certified Nutrition Consultant,
author of *Nourishing Hope for Autism*

"A food-writer and nutritionist who has turned her food-based misfortunes into health and real knowledge through education and experience, Mira Dessy will sit you down and tell you clearly how to, well, order your pantry: what to eat, what to buy, what to keep on hand, and how to apply your new understanding when you feed yourself and your family. Mira's friendly and conversational style disarms skepticism. Her tips offer easily-remembered nuggets of wisdom, and her Pantry Principle chart should guide your own pantry makeover. Mira's recipes made me want to run to the kitchen and cook them. A well-thumbed and thoroughly-read copy of Mira Dessy's *The Pantry Principle* should hold an honored place on the cookbook shelf of every person interested in the basics of food and good health."

— Beth Marshall, Web Designer and Artist, shares cooking with her spouse, Phil,
and plans to share Mira's wisdom with their adult daughter Jenn.

"Cleaning out the pantry is the perfect place to begin a journey towards healthy eating. *The Pantry Principle* does an excellent job of explaining the hidden ingredients lurking on grocery store shelves that stand between you and good health. Mira Dessy has created an indispensable guide to put your pantry and your health in great shape."

— Rebecca Katz, author of *The Longevity Kitchen: Satisfying Big-Flavor Recipes Featuring the Top 16 Age-Busting Power Foods*

Mira Dessy has written a indispensable handbook for people who want to eat real foods that nourish our brains and bodies, rather than gimmicky, artificially colored, flavored, and processed foods that make many people sick. If we all ate the way Mira recommends, we would have a much healthier population and planet. I hope we get there and this book is a great place to start.

— Aviva Goldfarb, Family Dinner Expert and
Founder of The Six O'Clock Scramble

"*The Pantry Principle* is a must have if you want to keep you and your family healthy!

If you think you know how to pick healthy foods for you and your family, you are in for a shock! Mira Dessy goes in depth to demystify the ingredients you glaze over in the grocery store and how they could be affecting your health or worse your child's health.

Learn the Good, the Bad and the Ugly on sweeteners, fats, additives, preservatives, colorings, genetically modified foods, organic foods, and more. It's all laid out in plain simple terms for you to understand. Add in awesome healthy recipes and then form it into your own Pantry Makeover with charts, and step-by-step action plans to create your own healthy pantry right in the book!

Get the best food bang for your buck with *The Pantry Principle*; a must have for everyone!"

— Karen Langston, Certified Holistic Nutritionist, specializing in Crohn's Disease

"*The Pantry Principle* is an easy-to-follow reference guide for anyone looking to give their pantry a healthy makeover. From step-by-step action plans, to comparison charts and a detailed recipe index, this book is a must have for every kitchen."

— Karen Roth, MS, CNC, Holistic Nutritionist, co-author of
I Married A Nutritionist: Things I've Learned That Every Guy Should Know

"Many people want to eat better, but don't know where to start. *The Pantry Principle* lays it all out so simply that anyone can make baby steps without feeling overwhelmed. Each chapter includes simple action steps to implement. You too can eat for health!"

— Heather Lionelle, Editor, Traditions Media and Publishing, LLC

"Mira took a personal nightmare and turned it into an opportunity for growth. Through her own education she improved her health, her family's health and if you read her book, your health.

The Pantry Principle offers basic information on everything from nutrition labels to ingredients and additives to healthy fats. I recommend reading Mira's book: it will help you obtain or maintain your good health."

— Patty James, M.S., C.N.C., DirectionFive Health, Founder and Director
Nutritionist/Chef/Writer, co-author of *More Vegetables, Please!*

The Pantry Principle

How to read the label and
understand what's really in your food

by Mira Dessy, NE

Foreword by Liz Lipski, PhD, CCN, CNS, CHN

Permission requests, speaking arrangements, and wholesale inquiries may be addressed to:

Versadia Press
10561 Blue Bell Drive
Willis, TX 77318

Printed in the United States of America

1st printing – 2013
2nd printing – 2017

ISBN: 978-0-9889357-0-9

EDITOR: DONNA MOSHER, SEGUE COMMUNICATIONS
ASSOCIATE EDITOR: HOLLY CASTER
COVER AND INTERIOR BOOK DESIGN: SUSAN B. GLATTSTEIN
AUTHOR PHOTO: LEE ANNA LOEHR, L.A. LOEHR PHOTOGRAPHY

Contact Information:
website: *www.The PantryPrinciple.net*
Facebook: *www.facebook.com/thepantryprinciple*
Twitter: *www.twitter.com/MiraDessy*

Disclaimer

The author of this book is not a doctor. The information in this book should not be considered medical advice and is not intended to treat, diagnose, prevent or cure any conditions, physical or otherwise. If you require medical advice or attention, please consult a physician or other health professional.

Information provided in this book has not been reviewed or approved by any federal, state, or local agency or healthcare group. Opinions expressed are solely those of the author and do not represent any particular individual or professional group.

ACKNOWLEDGEMENTS

This book owes thanks to many people; I couldn't have done what I did without their help, encouragement, and support. Grateful thanks are offered here for each and every one of them and all they contributed this project. I am richer for the gift of their presence.

First and foremost, to my wonderful husband, Steve, and our three fabulous daughters, Sasha, Veronica, and Diana, who have walked (and occasionally been dragged) along this path with me; your love and your belief in me sustains me.

To my wonderful friend Helene Purdy, the catalyst who started me down this path, I am forever in your debt for helping me find what I was meant to do in life.

To my mentors: Dr. Helayne Waldman who supported and cheered for me along the way. To Trudy Scott, whose kind words, amazing ideas, and continual encouragement have always been a blessing, I appreciate you.

For Dr. Liz Lipski who sets a shining example of what is possible, you are one of my personal heroes. To my many friends and colleagues at the National Association of Nutrition Professionals, I feel privileged to belong to such a great group of people.

And last, but certainly never least, I thank the outstanding team I was blessed to work with in the creation of this book. Donna Mosher is the best editor, idea-bouncer, and foodie friend anyone could want. Holly Caster is a talented, eagle-eyed associate editor, and my nsnbf. Susan Glattstein is a most amazing graphic designer, listener, creative force, and the best Aunt Susan there is.

Most of all, I owe an enormous debt of gratitude to the clients I have worked with over the years; you know who you are. Words cannot express how privileged I feel for the opportunity to work with each and every one of you. Your enthusiasm, curiosity, and commitment to better health inspired me to write this book. Thank you.

FORWARD

Most of the food we eat today would be unrecognizable to our ancestors. Food manufacturers can make more profit by creating "products" than by selling whole foods. As consumers, we love the convenience and taste of packaged foods. But is it in our best interest to do so? It's the life in food that gives us life. What we have come to call food is typically restructured, food-like substances that are stripped of most of their nutrients and life. These highly processed foods ultimately cheat our health. Many have been adulterated with chemicals that make us sick.

Early researchers, such as Albert Schweitzer and Weston Price, reported that people who ate traditional diets were free of cancer, diabetes, appendicitis, and heart disease. Today these diseases predominate in our society when one in every two men and one in every three women will develop cancer, when cardiovascular disease is the number one killer of women, where diabetes and metabolic syndrome are affecting children at earlier ages, and where it's expected that today's children will have shorter lifespans than their parents.

So what can you do? Current research indicates that even adding some natural foods back to the diets of indigenous people helps to prevent these diseases. Ultimately we are ALL indigenous people. So by moving to a more natural diet you may find that you feel more energetic, happier, or have normalized health issues that had bothered you.

This is true of Mira Dessy, the author of *The Pantry Principle*. Mira's health suffered, but as she began changing her lifestyle and the foods she ate, her body healed. Mira was inspired to learn more about nutrition by going back to school. She began going into people's homes and teaching them how to eat a more healthful diet. She took people through grocery stores helping them find healthier substitutions for the products they wanted to eat. She began teaching people how to cook and prepare simple and delicious meals at home.

Food today is confusing. Labeling is misleading. You are not alone if you can't figure out whether to buy free range, organic, vegetarian fed, or conventional eggs. This book helps to take the mystery out of shopping, food labeling, and whether ingredients are to be avoided or embraced. It teaches you how to replace foods that you typically eat with more healthful versions of the same foods. It's not about depriving yourself. The more you understand about food and nutrition, the easier it is to make positive changes in your diet. It's not about eating perfectly, but about making small improvements that can have far reaching results. By breaking down the information that you need to know across all categories of food and food additives Mira provides a straightforward, easy-to-follow resource that clearly defines what's really in your food.

As an example of how powerful a single nutritional change can be, I was teaching an eight week course at a university last summer. Several of the students decided to stop eating all refined sugar for the duration of the course. The results were dramatic. Several lost weight. One stopped having migraine headaches. Most experienced a surge of energy and clearer thinking. Several stopped being depressed.

Understanding the differences between complex and refined sugars is not always straightforward. In Chapter Five Mira clearly defines not only the different types of sugars but how they affect your metabolism and some of the deeper, negative health effects from overconsumption. She also provides a Sugar Action Plan giving you the support you need to make positive, healthy changes.

You are what you eat. Each cell in your body is comprised primarily of foods that you put into your mouth. With *The Pantry Principle* you can begin to make the journey towards health. It's filled with simple and delicious recipes and ideas for making simple shopping changes that can have big effects.

Enjoy,

Liz Lipski, PhD, CCN, CNS, CHN

Education Director of the Nutrition and Integrative Health Department
    Tai Sophia Institute, Laurel, MD

Author of *Digestive Wellness, Digestive Wellness for Children,*
    and *Leaky Gut Syndrome*

TABLE OF CONTENTS

My Story

I always prided myself on eating well and on feeding my family well, or at least what I thought was better than average. Not too much junk food, not much in the way of soda; our family ate lots of what I thought were healthy foods. I cooked almost every meal we ate. I made nearly all of our baked goods and preserves. We didn't eat out much. When we did we didn't really think too much about where we were going. I didn't read labels, I didn't think about non-food ingredients, I just cooked and fed us. I had no idea that I wasn't eating well for me or for my body.

My body started changing years before, as I say, I "got sick." I started experiencing severe stomach pain and bloating. After several office visits and numerous tests, my doctor told me I had irritable bowel syndrome (IBS). I was just thirty-three-years old! It didn't seem fair that this was happening to me. I tried a few different medications but didn't like the side effects, so I stopped, determined to "just live with it." It never dawned on me that my food could be the problem. No one ever talked to me about that.

After eight years of just living with it, I got *really* sick. It started with the dizziness. Sometimes the room seemed to slip sideways if I stood in one place too long or if I stood up too fast. Then I started having weakness in my limbs. I ignored it for a while, sure that I was somehow just being a wuss and that it would go away. But it didn't. I continued to have dizzy spells. When I finally went to the doctor, tests showed that I was severely anemic, drastically low on vitamin D, and my blood pressure was ridiculously low. I was put on prescription-strength iron supplements, 50,000 IU of vitamin D twice a week for eight weeks, and told to eat more salt. Taking that much vitamin D is serious business. The Vitamin D Council suggests as much as 5,000 IU per day if you are not getting adequate sun exposure. At 50,000 IU you don't take it every day, and you have to go in for regular blood tests to make sure you don't wind up with toxic levels of vitamin D in your system. There was no satisfactory explanation for why my levels were so low. And still no one talked to me about my food. So I took the supplements and thought I felt a little better, but I was still struggling.

I also started having other symptoms that I didn't want to tell anyone about. My IBS appeared to be getting worse. I frequently had cramps after I ate, and sometimes they were so painful that I was doubled over on the toilet immediately after eating. I felt bloated and alternated between diarrhea and constipation on a regular basis. I also noticed a white coating on my stools (I didn't know it was mucous; I just thought it was odd). And, as embarrassing as this is to admit, I started having fecal accidents. I was so ashamed that I couldn't bring myself to talk to anyone about it. I hid it from everyone: my husband, my family, my doctor, my co-workers, everyone.

One day I saw blood in the toilet. That was it; in a panic I called the doctor's office to schedule an appointment. Practically whispering into the phone, I simply told them I had seen blood. They were very laid back about the situation and told me I probably had hemorrhoids but to come in and they would examine me. The physician's assistant who saw me confirmed that I had blood in my stool. I didn't tell her about the accidents because I was so humiliated by it. That visit, however, led to a consultation with a gastroenterologist. When he asked pointed questions about my symptoms, I finally confessed everything. He sent me for a colonoscopy. The results revealed that, after nearly a decade of being diagnosed with IBS, I didn't have IBS. I had ulcerative colitis.

As part of my treatment plan it was suggested that I consider dietary changes for a short period of time so that my digestive system could heal. I felt so much better in just a few days! I enthusiastically embraced my new diet and began to read and learn everything I could about it, although there did not appear to be a lot of information readily available.

Even though my gut felt better and my symptoms were improving, overall I got worse. I was perpetually dizzy and felt weak. I also began to feel very overwhelmed when doctor after doctor couldn't find anything wrong with me (besides what they had already identified, which apparently should not have been enough to make me feel this bad). I began to become very sensitive to smells. If people around me were wearing heavy perfumes I felt nauseous. I got a headache just walking through the detergent aisle at the grocery store.

At this point I stopped working. Although I did not leave my job specifically for health reasons, that departure turned out to be a blessing in disguise. In my declining condition I would not have been able to continue to perform well at that position. At my absolute worst I spent most of my time lying on the sofa. I had perhaps one or two good hours a day when I could make dinner or try to stuff a load of laundry into the machine. Driving my kids to various activities was torture and exhausting. If I walked up a flight of stairs, I literally had to lie down at the top for a while before I could go any further.

The turning point came after two doctors' visits in one week. By this time I was seeing five or six doctors on a regular basis, and I was taking more pills than I care to remember. My rheumatologist told me that he wanted to put me on a particular medication, but he was pretty sure my endocrinologist wouldn't approve, so he wasn't going to do it. I was angry. If he thought that was what I needed, why didn't he just call her up and talk to her about it? And why on earth would he tell me that if he didn't intend to advocate for me? Later in the week I went to see a new doctor who, after hearing my tale of woe, said to me, "Well, Mrs. Dessy, you are getting older." As I drove home I got more than mad. I became furious. I was only forty-two-years old. I realized at that point that he had written me off. Perhaps all the doctors had, and this was not an acceptable situation.

As soon as I got home I called my insurance company, and I read them the riot act. In hindsight, I feel sorry for the woman who took my call, because I was on a tirade, yelling at someone whose only job was to answer the phone. I wish there was some way I could go back and apologize for my rudeness. As I was screaming out my frustrations, I pointed out to her that the insurance company was spending huge sums of money on doctors and medications and, according to this last doctor, there was no end in sight. I was angry that the doctors wouldn't talk to each other, and I felt as if I was being treated like a product rather than a person. I was overwhelmed that after more than a year of treatment I wasn't getting better, and I felt that no one cared. After I finally wound down enough to ask her what the insurance company planned to do to correct this situation, she offered me an executive checkup at a major national hospital. I was stunned. I didn't even know such an option existed. I grabbed at it with both hands.

An executive checkup, I learned, is a pretty amazing thing. First of all you are assigned a "medical concierge" who makes all of your appointments for you, holds your hand in the waiting room if needed, makes sure you know how to get anywhere you need to go, and is available at the drop of a hat. Then you are assigned a "gateway doctor" who receives the reports from the other doctors and who heads up your team. In a period of four days I saw a whole host of doctors who poked and prodded, who asked a lot of questions, and, most importantly, who listened. I came home with a lot of new information, some new treatment plans, and a new, powerful determination to be an active participant in my own health care.

I started by making further changes to our food and reading everything I could get my hands on. I also learned more about digestion and began to work harder to support my digestive process. The more I learned, the more I wanted to know. In my reading I began to learn how the ingredients in food are more important than I had previously thought. All the artificial ingredients, the chemical soup that I had been putting into my body, the non-food items that I had been eating, all of these I believe had slowly contributed to the decline of my health.

Slowly, step by step, I began to remove various foods from our diet (because if I was going to eat this way, so was my family). I started with those with the obvious chemicals, the ones that I could easily identify. I also began to pay attention to more than just what the food was— meat, dairy, produce, and so forth—and began to focus on the *quality* of the food we were eating. This process took a long time. I realized this was not going to be a quick fix. Although I was initially frustrated, a good friend pointed out that it had taken a very long time for me to get to the point where I was. To be successful I needed to make small, achievable changes, one step at a time. And I needed to avoid becoming overwhelmed with what I wasn't doing, and to focus on how far I had come in successfully changing our diet.

At a certain point I made the decision to go back to school and study holistic nutrition. I became a Certified Nutrition Educator, graduating with honors, and began a new career, one that allowed me to help not just my family and me but also to support others and help them to fully understand the connection between their food and their health.

Today, I am happy to report that I am healthy. I feel great. I do not require daily pharmaceuticals to manage my condition, and I have successfully implemented a wide variety of changes to our diet that are more supportive of our health. In making small, focused, sustainable changes we have been able to continue to eat well, and I believe we are all healthier for it.

This is why I wrote this book. The idea for it has been germinating for a long time, starting in 2006. It began as I started teaching people about healthy, whole-food eating: how to cook with whole grains; tasty ways to add more fresh foods to their diet; and how to make changes in their nutritional patterns, their kitchens, and their lives.

One of my first classes was called "The Poison Pantry: three things you should not eat and why." Needless to say, there were more than three things on that list but it was enough to get everyone's attention. No one likes the idea that their pantry may be making their family sick. People were startled to learn what was really in their food. Through my classes, talking about all of these factors, I was helping them learn which choices were better. I educated them and helped them to navigate the sometimes confusing and overwhelming array of non-nutritional choices available. I equipped them with the knowledge they needed to take back control of their pantries, their diets, and their health.

As I was teaching the class I began to realize that simply talking to people about what to eat, what not to eat, and why wasn't enough. I needed to get to the heart of the matter. I started offering a service I called a "Pantry Party," in which I would visit their homes to go through their pantry with them. I brought handouts and provided one-on-one attention for their specific pantry. The purpose was to help them better understand what they were eating and how to improve their choices and their health. We started with the foods that were in the pantry, items that they were already eating and obviously liked. They were learning how to still eat many of their favorite foods, but making better choices. They were also learning to understand why these changes were important. The pantry parties were fun, and folks were thrilled to have me come into their homes and to show them where they could make positive, beneficial improvements to their food storage systems and their health.

I clearly remember one family where the mom insisted that everyone in the house, both parents and the children, participate in the experience. Dad stood by the front door with a hangdog expression on his face when I entered the house. "You're going to tell me I can't eat anything I like," he grumbled. I assured him that my role was to help him better understand his choices, not to play food police. Step by step, we worked together so everyone could understand exactly what was in the food. I gave them information that empowered them to make choices that would better support their diet and their health. By the end of the visit the dad was the one who was most enthusiastically diving into the closet, pulling out various items and asking me to explain the what, why, and wherefore of each one. We were able to come up with good substitutes for those things that needed to leave the house, modifications that were tasty and yet did not leave any member of this family feeling deprived in any way.

As time went by, I focused even more on helping people create a healthy pantry. I realized we needed to start at the source: where they were buying their food. Occasionally gathering small crowds of interested bystanders eavesdropping for free advice, I began taking individual clients with their shopping lists through the grocery stores of their choice. Because we knew what they wanted to eat, we could focus on understanding those items and how to improve on their choices. Walking through the store, they were learning how to read and understand a nutrition label. They learned how to assess and understand the ingredients in the food they were buying and how to make changes for their health in a supportive, encouraging way. One couple said it was "a real eye-opener that changed our whole way of shopping for food. Now even our two sons, ages 11 and 14, are avid label readers." Another person enthusiastically declared that learning this information made her feel good about herself and her commitment to her health. It was a gratifying and enriching experience for me as well to know that I was helping these people make positive changes, giving them skills and knowledge that they could use for the rest of their lives.

As people began to talk to their friends and family members further away, it became apparent that I could travel only so far to help folks. After all, if your pantry is in Sherman, Connecticut, and I'm in The Woodlands, Texas, it's not going to work very well.

With the encouragement of my family, friends, and happy clients, I turned my efforts into creating this book for people who cannot work with me in person. I wanted to share my knowledge in a good stand-alone reference for folks to understand what's in their food. I wanted to teach them how to make better choices for themselves and their loved ones.

You now hold in your hands my compiled lectures, handouts, some great recipes, and other resource information for a holistically healthy pantry and how to provide clean, healthy foods for you and your loved ones. I am grateful for your purchase of this book, I'm thrilled for your desire to make better choices in how you fuel your body, and I wish you all the best on your journey toward better health.

Eat well, be well,

Mira Dessy
The Woodlands, TX

Introduction

From the days of hunter-gathers to modern shoppers attempting to decipher the complexity of products on food shelves, the way we procure our food has changed dramatically. But our need for proper nourishment remains the same. Processed food, fast food, adulterated and chemically enhanced foods make navigating the stocking of our pantries with healthy foods a truly mystifying chore.

In the US, although we have legislation governing what is allowed and not allowed in various products, many of us have become very disconnected from our food. We don't know where it comes from, and we don't know what's really in it. I bet you're like most people: when you walk into a grocery store, you think that all of the edible-appearing products on the shelves are food. The truth is that many of them are not! Many of these items contain ingredients that have the potential to be harmful. It hasn't always been that way.

Food started off as a fairly simple, plain affair. It began with meat, poultry, and fish that were hunted plus edible roots, nuts, greens, and berries that were gathered seasonally. This formed the basis of the prehistoric diet. The advent of cooking, possibly as early as 500,000 BCE, marginally improved nutrition, as heat is known to break down the fibers in many foods as well as to release nutrients in some foods. Over the millennia food preparation techniques evolved slowly, with bread not making a consistent appearance until somewhere around the 4th century BCE.

As humans became less nomadic, food changed and was modified. New foodstuffs were discovered, and different preparation methods arose. Along with the advent of the pantry, food storage methods were developed, mostly involving smoking and salting, drying, and a fair amount of preservation through encasing foods in fat. By the late 1700s preservation methods included heating meats, fruits, vegetables, jams, and even milk in corked glass jars. By the early 1800s tinned, or canned, foods had been developed (although the can opener was not developed until 1855). Soon canned foods became widely available and the practice of purchasing foods for longer-term storage or travel took off. Also around this time food substitutes began to creep into our diet; margarine was invented in the late 1860s when Napoleon III sponsored a contest seeking butter substitutes.

The concept of refrigeration most likely appeared around 600 BCE in China when winter ice was cut and stored for summer use. Ice-making machines were patented in the 1830s with widespread use of refrigeration beginning in 1850 making food storage and long-term preservation possible. The first known example of a major use of refrigeration was a banquet held in 1873 where guests supped from meats and fish harvested and frozen six months prior to the meal.

Food, especially processed food, has often been changed in some way — by the consumer to store it for long-term use and by the producer to try to make more money from the product. Food adulteration became commonplace during the mid-19th century when expensive or rare items were contaminated, bulked up, or counterfeited with cheaper ingredients. Pepper was bulked up with mustard husks or pea flour, wooden balls were sold as nutmeg, and bread was contaminated with alum to make it look white. Even tea was bulked up with dried ash tree leaves or with leftover tea leaves which were dried, treated with a stiffening solution, and then colored with black lead before being resold as fresh. Nor were these the only additives used. Some preparations were potentially lethal with producers using bitter almond, copper salts, or sulphate of iron.

In 1875 the first legislation was passed to protect the purity of food products. While legislation and oversight has been greatly expanded since then, there are still examples of food adulteration, sometimes with fatal results. Recent horrifying examples include melamine, a waste product of the construction industry, added to milk powder, which increases the appearance of protein but can lead to kidney failure when ingested. Another recently discovered adulteration was that of fake rice, which was found to be made from potatoes and plastic resin. It is important to know that both of these examples originated in China; however with the advent of a global food supply it makes understanding what's really in your pantry even more important.

Even though legislation generally protects us against illegal food substances, and many things in our food are recognized by government agencies as "Generally Recognized As Safe" (GRAS), evidence is showing many of these GRAS items to be either unsafe or at the very least not nutritious healthy food options. We find ourselves being seduced by the pretty pictures on the box or the marketing claims by the manufacturer. We don't really know what's in our food, trusting that if they are selling it we can eat it.

This book is a reference guide to change that. It is a way for you to take back control of your pantry and your food source. In reading and using this book you will learn how to identify those items that are not contributing anything to your nutrition and certainly not to your health nor that of your loved ones.

What you hold in your hands is not a "read it once and you are done" type of book. The information contained between its covers encompasses a wide range of food-related subjects. By opening this book you have embarked on a journey to make positive changes in your food supply and your health. But these changes will not happen overnight; this will be an ongoing journey. My suggestion is that you read this book front to back so that you know what is involved in understanding the complexity of products at the grocery store.

Once you have read the book, you will begin your journey toward the Pantry Principle, toward building a healthy food source in your home. Start with the Seven Simple Rules in Chapter One. Then in Chapter Two you'll learn How To Read A Nutrition Label. If nothing else, this is the most important skill you can teach yourself when it comes to purchasing manufactured or prepared foods. Then choose one area at a time where you wish to make further changes. Re-read whichever chapter you want to work on. This book is your study guide: tag, underline, or highlight the information that is of most interest to you. Make notes for yourself as you begin to prune items from your pantry and to watch out for undesirable ingredients at the grocery store. When you are confident that you have mastered one area, you can move on to another. This is a reference book that you can come back to over and over again.

It may seem confusing and overwhelming at first. You may struggle a little with looking for healthier alternatives for the products that you are used to. But if you stick with it you will find yourself gaining knowledge and confidence as you go along. With the help of this book you will master this information and create a positive change in your home.

If along the way you discover that you have made a mistake and purchased a food product that is not in accordance with the Pantry Principle, don't worry. We all make mistakes. As long as it is unopened you can take it back to the grocery store. If they question you about why you are returning the item, tell them honestly that you did not realize that the item contains an ingredient that you cannot eat.

I would like to share a personal story about grocery shopping. I don't like okra. Now, I live in the South where that borders on heretical, but there is something about it that just does not appeal to me. I did eventually discover, however, that I like okra pickled. So when I saw a new product prominently displayed on the shelves at my grocery store, pickled okra, I eagerly grabbed the jar, added it to my cart, and continued shopping. When I got home I checked the label and was startled to discover that it contained polysorbate 80 and artificial coloring. I was disappointed, but needless to say I took it back to the grocery store.

There are two pieces of information that I would like you to take from this story. The first is that mistakes happen, especially when we're in a hurry, or we are distracted. Even if we know what we are doing, we can overlook something. The second is to always read the label. I truly try to read the labels at the store to save myself the time and inconvenience of purchasing and then returning a product. But if I do not take the time to read the label in the grocery store, I always read it, especially for new products, before it goes into my pantry. This is a habit that I highly encourage you to learn.

The word pantry originated in the 13th century as an Anglo-Saxon derivation of the French word *paneterie*, meaning "bread room" and was the office of the servant in charge of bread (common definitions seem to indicate that the words for bread and food at this point in time were used interchangeably). As far as I am concerned, anywhere that you store food to hold it until you are ready to prepare it for consumption qualifies as part of your pantry. This includes the traditional food closet, the kitchen cupboards, the fruit bowl on the counter, the refrigerator, the freezer, the extra freezer in the garage or basement, a box under your bed, even the closet under the stairs. If you store food there, it counts as a pantry space. I don't differentiate between different types of food, either. With the advent of warehouse shopping clubs we have increased what and how much we buy. No longer purchasing just for everyday eating, we do not shop on a daily basis. Many families purchase perishables on a weekly basis, non-perishables less frequently, and then buy food for long-term storage or emergencies. It is all part of your pantry, your household food system. Because this is your food source, what you feed yourself and your family, you want the healthiest choices available in your pantry.

Welcome to *The Pantry Principle*. Your journey to improved health is about to begin!

CHAPTER ONE

Seven Simple Rules

Most people assume when they buy groceries that everything available in the store, everything they are purchasing to eat, is food. Unfortunately this is not the case. Unless you stick to the perimeter of your grocery store when you shop, where the "real" food is, you will generally be considering processed food for purchase. If it is in a box, in a can, or in a jar and has a list of ingredients on the label, it has been processed. This means the food has been changed from its natural state. Manufacturers process food for a number of reasons, including to extend shelf life, for convenience of preparation, to enhance taste, to boost sales, etc.

Here is a simple way to know if food is processed: If it is in your pantry, it probably has been processed!

Now, that doesn't mean it shouldn't be in your pantry. My pantry is well stocked with jars, cans, and even a few boxes of packaged foods. It just means you need to read to label to learn if the ingredients are safe and truly healthy for you to eat. Now that we know how to read labels, let's learn a little more about what we're looking for.

There are many additives, preservatives, and other chemicals that adulterate our food. These chemicals not only reduce the nutritional value of what we are eating; for many people the chemical accumulation can cause illness or otherwise deplete our health.

My friend and mentor, Dr. Helayne Waldman, has an analogy which I believe clearly illustrates the concept of why we need to pay attention to our food. When architects go to school to learn their craft, they don't just learn the principles of design. They also learn about the building blocks: bricks, mortar, steel, concrete, and all the different elements that are required to create a strong a beautiful building. Unfortunately we don't learn these things when it comes to our food, but it's just as important for us to understand the building blocks of what creates a strong and healthy body. Those foods that we eat get turned into our cells, which in turn support, nourish, and grow our blood, skin, bones, muscles, etc. By using good building materials, or food, we support a stronger system — our body.

It is, however, important to remember that implementing these rules (and indeed all of the information in this book) is not meant to be accomplished immediately. It would be very overwhelming, and quite possibly unsustainable, to throw everything out, start from scratch with rules and ideas you don't fully understand, and then move forward with never a glance back. Because we are learning new information while changing habits and palates, this process, takes time to incorporate into your shopping, storage, cooking, and eating routines. Many of the foods you may be giving up are actually addictive; this means that it also takes time to retrain your palate. [BBC. 2003] [Lenoir, et al. 2007]

These changes need to be implemented slowly and consistently. Pick the changes you can easily start (I suggest you start with the seven rules that follow) and then make modifications and improvements a little at a time. Remember that this book is a reference book, meant to be utilized over and over as you learn to make health-supporting changes.

It is also important that you not get overwhelmed with whatever you think you are not doing. There is a health condition called orthorexia. The dictionary defines it as "a disorder characterized by a morbid obsession with eating healthy foods only." The object is not to become so hyper-focused on your food that you don't enjoy it or that you cannot eat anything that does not "fit" the rules. The goal is to make decisions that support your health and your body while at the same time making informed choices about your food. Remember that each change you make, each decision about your food, is more than you were doing before and is done at a level which is comfortable and achievable for you. Baby steps, taking things one at a time, will be more sustainable in the long run. Recall Aesop's fable of the tortoise and the hare: slow and steady wins the race.

To be healthy we need to feed our bodies healthy choices. This means clean foods that nourish and support our health. The basic principles of keeping a healthy pantry are the seven simple rules that follow. Specific information relating to different sections of what you might find at the grocery store (such as purchasing organic foods or understanding dairy products) are found in the other chapters of this book. By following these seven simple rules that make up the mainstay of the Pantry Principle, you become a better shopper. By learning to really understand what's in your food you can become not only a great shopper, but a champion for health.

Here are the seven simple rules. While there are exceptions to some of the rules, these seven form a strong basis to help you navigate the aisles at the grocery store:

1. ***If you don't know what it is, don't eat it.*** After all, do you really know what butyl formate is? Probably not. If you research it you'll find that it is a synthetic flavoring additive made from formic acid. Now do you understand what it is? My answer is still no, not really. So it clearly doesn't make sense to eat it.

2. ***If it has a number, don't eat it.*** Food does not grow by numbers. Anything with a number on it, such as polysorbate 60 or red #2, is a manufactured ingredient and therefore not a whole food. This means it is not something you want to put in your body.

3. ***If it has four or more syllables, don't eat it.*** Real food, whole food, is simple and straightforward. Kale, milk, banana, eggplant, Brazil nut, all fall into this rule. Whole foods such as macadamia are an exception, but this rule cuts out a lot of processed foods.

4. ***If you can't pronounce it, don't eat it.*** This would include words like acetaldehyde diisoamyl acetyal, a long name for a synthetic flavoring. Or phenylpropyl, part of different names for other synthetic flavorings. These artificial ingredients do not belong in your pantry or in your body. Exceptions would include foods like acai (ah-sigh-ee) or quinoa (keen-wa) which are whole foods.

5. ***If an ingredient ends in a-t-e, don't e-a-t it.*** This rule of thumb works well for avoiding certain artificial ingredients such as methyl acetate. Made from acetic acid, methyl acetate is used

as a flavoring. Unfortunately it is also used to dissolve some oils and resins. Given the latter why would you want to eat it? Obviously this would not apply to a whole food such as pomegranate, however, overall this rule is a good one and very easy to remember.

6. *If it says "enriched", don't eat it.* We talk about this in Chapter Two; enriched means the food has been stripped of some, or many, of its naturally occurring components. Enriched wheat flour is a prime example and found in many products such as bread, crackers, and cookies.

7. *If an ingredient is all capital letters, don't eat it.* While many of us remember alphabet soup from our childhood, we shouldn't be eating ingredients that consist only of letters and which don't spell a real word. BHT, TBHQ, EDTA: these things are not food and should not be in your pantry.

In order to make it easier at the grocery store I've included a wallet card below. Simply make a copy and then cut it out and take it with you. This will help you to remember the rules of the Pantry Principle until they become a healthy habit, something you remember without thinking about it.

READ THE INGREDIENTS:

- Do you have to look it up?
- Does it have a number?
- Does it have four or more syllables?
- Is it unpronounceable?
- Does it end in a-t-e?
- Is it enriched?
- Is it all capital letters, not words?

If you answered yes to any of these, don't eat it!

ThePantryPrinciple.net

Note: There are a few exceptions; think critically about your choices.

Following these seven simple rules can help you become a good, healthy shopper. These straightforward ideas will go a long way toward helping you avoid a lot of ingredients that you do not want to feed yourself or your loved ones.

Now that you understand the basic rules, let's take it up a notch and move on to becoming a champion at the grocery store.

CHAPTER TWO

How to Read a Nutrition Label

The first lesson of stocking a healthy pantry is to learn just what ingredients are in the food you buy. You are already a savvy grocery shopper, or you would not be reading this book. You already know the importance of whole grains, you want to avoid eating trans-fats, and you want to minimize your consumption of sugar. But do you really know what is in the food—particularly the packaged food—you are buying?

Just because a food's package says it is good for you doesn't mean it is. Consider PepsiCo's "Smartspot," Kraft's "Sensible Solutions," Sara Lee's "Nutritional Spotlight." These labels pretend to help you make such decisions as whether baked potato chips are healthier than fried. There is a lot more to learn from a package than that!

We're going to start with what you might consider an unnecessary, or challenging, or just plain boring topic: How to read a nutrition label. You will learn how to find out what is in processed food. You will learn and how manufacturers try to conceal certain ingredients you want to avoid. You will learn how to pass up those pretty packages that claim they contain healthful foods. And by the end of the chapter, you will be able to walk into any grocery store with confidence that you can choose precisely the foods you want your family to eat.

One of the challenges facing many people when they are in the grocery store is understanding the label on the package. Some people are so overwhelmed by the label that they bypass it altogether. Or perhaps they only look at one or two pieces of information. I cannot stress enough how very important it is to learn to read the label. That point is so important that I'm going to say it again. To make healthy choices for yourself and your family you **must** learn to **read the label**.

In the early 13th century, the king of England issued the first food regulatory law, which prohibited bakers from mixing ground peas and beans into bread dough. In the United States the government has been regulating the food industry since Lincoln established the Bureau of Chemistry, the predecessor of the Food and Drug Administration (FDA). In 1990, Congress passed the Nutrition Labeling and Education Act, requiring that all packaged foods show nutrition labeling and that all health claims for foods be consistent with terms defined by the Secretary of Health and Human Services. The Center for Food Safety and Applied Nutrition now oversees the safe and accurate labeling of almost all food products sold in the United States.

What is on the label has undergone a number of changes since labels were first mandated. Currently there are two categories of information to be found on the label: the mandatory information and the voluntary information. Mandatory information is required by law and includes the total number of calories, information about fat (including calories from fat, total fats, saturated fat, and trans-fats), cholesterol, sodium, total carbohydrates, protein, sugars, several micronutrients (specifically vitamins A, C, calcium, and iron), and dietary fiber (but not the fiber breakdown).

Because voluntary information is not required, some manufacturers leave it out of the labeling while others choose to include it. The information often displayed can include a further breakdown of the calories from saturated fat, the amount of monounsaturated fats and polyunsaturated fats, potassium, the amounts of both soluble and insoluble fiber, any sugar alcohols, the amount of vitamin A as beta carotene, and any other essential vitamins and minerals. If a manufacturer makes a claim regarding any of the voluntary information such as stating a product is "high in beta carotene," that section becomes mandatory on the label. It is also required to display the information if a food is fortified or enriched with anything from the voluntary categories. For example, if orange juice is fortified with calcium, the amount of calcium must then be clearly displayed on the nutrition label.

Fortified means nutrients have been added that are not normally part of that food; such as calcium in orange juice.
Enriched means nutrients lost in processing have been put back into the item; such as some of the B vitamins in wheat flour.

Currently there is pressure from organizations such as the Center for Science in the Public Interest (CSPI) to revise the label further and make it more consumer-friendly. These changes would include greater emphasis on highlighting calories, fats, sugars, cholesterol, and sodium. There is also a push to clearly identify true fiber, something that is not obvious on the current label. [CSPI, 2009] True fiber simply means fiber that comes from whole foods—beans, whole grains, fruits, and vegetables—rather than chemically added fibers such as maltodextrin.

Food labeling can be very misleading and difficult to understand. Unfortunately, if consumers do not really know what they are looking at or understand the information that is presented, they can often choose something which looks healthy, but ultimately isn't. One example was the short-lived Smart Choices food labeling system from 2009, which was supported by a number of manufacturers including Kraft, Pepsi, Unilever, and Kellogg. Essentially the system gave a large green check on the front of the box, signifying a "seal of approval" to products that met the nutritional guidelines.

It should come as no surprise to anyone that the companies who supported Smart Choices labeling gave their products high marks. For example Kellogg's Froot Loops cereal was given a check even though the first ingredient in the cereal is sugar. This information is usually present only if the manufacturer thinks it presents some sort of positive spin on their product. By prominently displaying a self-awarded "seal of approval," no doubt manufacturers were hoping consumers would purchase the product without examining the contents listed on the nutrition label.

Not only manufacturers, but retailers have tried to get into the labeling game. In February 2012 Wal-Mart announced it would begin using its own labeling system called "Great For You." Unfortunately just as manufacturers awarded themselves good marks for their own labeling, there exists a strong chance that retailers such as Wal-Mart will do the same, especially when it comes to their own in-store brands. To further complicate the issue of labeling, in June 2012 Disney announced its own system, as well as advertising standards for Disney Channel promotion, which they would implement on Disney-branded foods. This is a form of nutri-washing, a method where a company may appear to be making good health choices for the benefit of their consumers. The companies can and do use health concerns as a means of promoting not only their own brands but as a way to try to build further brand loyalty. However, when the issue is examined more deeply, it becomes clear that these labeling efforts are often used to try to direct sales rather than to serve as an educational tool for the consumer. This new, corporate-directed labeling scheme also provides the potential for Disney to use this label as a way to control products that may want to obtain the Disney brand.

Rather than being seduced by front-of-package labeling claims or bold-print partial truths, you need to learn how to read nutrition labels and understand the information presented there. That information will allow you to make better, more balanced choices based on a clear understanding of what is actually in your food.

NUTRITION FACTS

In order to understand a nutrition label, let's go through one step by step. For the purposes of this exercise I have chosen a simple box of macaroni and cheese, something that is found in most pantries.

The items at the top of the label are referred to as the Nutrition Facts.

Let's look at some of the facts. Starting at the top of the label, it is important to note how many servings are in the container. Frequently what might be considered a small container will actually have two or more servings in it. This means that if you consume the entire container you will need to multiply all of the nutritional information — calories,

---

Nutrition Facts

Serving Size 2.5 oz
(70g / about 1/3 Box)
(Makes about 1 cup)
Servings Per Container about 3

Amount Per Serving	As Packaged	As Prepared
Calories	250	410
Calories From Fat	20	160

	%Daily Value**	
Total Fat 2g*	3%	26%
Saturated Fat 1g	5%	20%
Trans Fat 0g		
Cholesterol 5mg	2%	3%
Sodium 570mg	24%	30%
Total Carbohydrate 50g	17%	17%
Dietary Fiber 2g	8%	8%
Sugars 8g		
Protein 9g		

Vitamin A	0%	15%
Vitamin C	0%	0%
Calcium	10%	15%
Iron	10%	10%

* Amount in Box. Preparation with Margarine and 2% Reduced Fat Milk adds 15g total fat (3g sat fat, 4g trans fat), 5mg cholesterol, 140mg sodium, 2g carbohydrate (2g sugars), and 1g protein.

** Percent Daily Values are based on a 2,000 calorie diet. Your daily values may be higher or lower depending on your calorie needs:

		Calories:	2,000	2,500
Total Fat	Less than		65g	80g
Sat Fat	Less than		20g	25g
Cholest	Less than		300mg	300mg
Sodium	Less than		2400mg	2400mg
Total Carb			300g	375g
Dietary Fiber			25g	30g

INGREDIENTS: ENRICHED MACARONI PRODUCT (WHEAT FLOUR, NIACIN, FERROUS SULFATE [IRON], THIAMIN MONONITRATE [VITAMIN B1], RIBOFLAVIN [VITAMIN B2], FOLIC ACID); CHEESE BLEND (WHEY, MODIFIED FOOD STARCH, SALT, MILKFAT, MILK PROTEIN CONCENTRATE, CONTAINS LESS THAN 2% OF SODIUM TRIPOLYPHOSPHATE, CELLULOSE GEL, CELLULOSE GUM, CITRIC ACID, SODIUM PHOSPHATE, CALCIUM PHOSPHATE, LACTIC ACID, YELLOW 5, YELLOW 6, ENZYMES, CHEESE CULTURE)

CONTAINS: WHEAT, MILK.

KRAFT FOODS GLOBAL, INC.
NORTHFIELD, IL 60093-2753 USA

fat, sugars, protein, and so forth — by the number of servings in the container to get the true numbers.

Most people don't take the time to look at the serving size. If they do, they may not take the time to do the math. If Brand A claims that ½ cup is 120 calories and Brand B claims that ¾ cup is 180 calories which one is lower in calories? Additionally many of us do not understand how much or how little a serving size really is. Do we measure out a half-cup or do we "eyeball" it? If we're being honest, most of us will confess that we simply pour or serve until it "looks right" and consider that the serving size. What we serve ourselves, the amount we choose to eat, is considered a portion. There are no standard portion sizes, which are frequently considerably larger than a serving. This means when eating a portion, most people are actually consuming more calories, in some cases far more, than they think they are. The manufacturer-listed serving size often is not a true measure of what the consumer considers to be a reasonable serving. For example, a 20-ounce drink may claim to have two servings when most consumers drink the entire bottle. The label on a 6-ounce can of tuna fish may say it contains 2.5 servings, but many people consider one can a single serving.

As to the ½ cup versus ¾ cup question above? The answer is they both have 60 calories per ¼ cup, so they are for all intents and purposes equal, at least as far as caloric count. Using our maccaroni and cheese label as an example, an entire box leaves you consuming around 750 calories, mostly from fat and carbohydrates.

After calories, most people look at the fat, cholesterol, and sodium content. The "% Daily Value" (DV) column to the right refers to the percentage of daily requirements for the listed item. In other words, the 2 grams of fat in that one serving of macaroni and cheese provides 3 percent of the fat that you need for the entire day. This does not include added fat from butter and/or milk which, as the label states, if prepared as directed could be 26 percent of the fat for an entire day. Remember this is <u>per serving</u> not per box. It is important to note that these percentages are based on a 2,000-calorie diet. If you do not need to consume 2,000 calories a day (or if you are Michael Phelps and require 12,000 calories a day when you are in training), you are going to have to do some math to figure out what your actual needs are.

Given our example of eating the entire box (about three servings) prepared as directed, you would consume approximately 78 percent of your daily value for fat, 9 percent for cholesterol, and 90 percent for sodium. Again, that's if you ate 2,000 calories a day. If you require only 1,800 calories a day, the percentages go up.

Notice that there is no daily requirement for sugar; this box contains 8 grams per serving. Unfortunately we have become addicted to sugar in this country, and we consume far too much of it. It is very important to look at the amount of sugar even though there is no DV listed. Eating too much sugar can have a negative effect on your health as the excess is converted to adipose, or fat, tissue. How much is too much? The American Heart Association recommends that women consume no more than 100 calories per day in added sugars. That's about six teaspoons. For men the recommendation is no more than 150 calories, or nine teaspoons. [AHA. 2009] Hold on to that thought, we'll discuss sugar and sweeteners in Chapter Five.

Other challenges to understanding the nutrition label are the items that appear to indicate they equal zero. I call this "Mystery Math." Many people do not realize that federal guidelines allow a manufacturer to claim that there is 0 percent of an ingredient (such as trans fatty acids, or "trans-fats") if the total value is less than .5 grams *per serving.*

Using trans-fats as an example, this is where you need to understand what is on the label and what is in the ingredients.

Trans-fats are fats that have been hydrogenated or partially hydrogenated in order to stay solid at room temperature — look for the words hydrogenated or partially hydrogenated in the ingredients section of the label.

If labeling laws allow for a less than .5 grams serving to be labeled as zero and yet trans-fats appear in the ingredients list, you are going to be consuming them. Even though the trans-fats may be less than .5 grams per serving, if you eat three servings of that product, you've consumed a potential 1.49 grams of trans-fats.

Why is this important? Many doctors consider trans-fats to be the worst type of fat, because it both raises your "bad" (LDL) cholesterol and lowers your "good" (HDL) cholesterol. Many people want to avoid trans-fats, so they read the label. When they see "0g trans-fats," they feel confident they are choosing a product without trans-fat. Maybe. Maybe not. So you can see why I call this type of labeling Mystery Math.

Nothing on our macaroni and cheese label example is a trans-fat, meaning the fat is not hydrogenated or partially hydrogenated, so we do not need to calculate it or watch out for it.

UNDERSTANDING INGREDIENTS

This brings us to the next part of the label, the ingredients list. Many people skip the ingredients, relying instead on the front of the package to tell them about the item they are purchasing. We'll discuss the front of the package in just a moment.

INGREDIENTS: ENRICHED MACARONI PRODUCT (WHEAT FLOUR, NIACIN, FERROUS SULFATE [IRON], THIAMIN MONONITRATE [VITAMIN B1], RIBOFLAVIN [VITAMIN B2], FOLIC ACID); CHEESE BLEND (WHEY, MODIFIED FOOD STARCH, SALT, MILKFAT, MILK PROTEIN CONCENTRATE, CONTAINS LESS THAN 2% OF SODIUM TRIPOLYPHOSPHATE, CELLULOSE GEL, CELLULOSE GUM, CITRIC ACID, SODIUM PHOSPHATE, CALCIUM PHOSPHATE, LACTIC ACID, YELLOW 5, YELLOW 6, ENZYMES, CHEESE CULTURE)
CONTAINS: WHEAT, MILK.

The higher up in the list an ingredient is, the more of that ingredient there is in the package. For our macaroni and cheese label listed above, the first ingredient is enriched macaroni product.

Too often manufacturers do not want to call attention to the primary ingredient in a product. Would you be inclined to buy what you think is a healthy product if the first ingredient listed on the label is sugar? Probably not. One way manufacturers try to keep a category of ingredients such as sugar from appearing too high on the list is to use several sources of the same ingredient. For example, if the label lists evaporated cane juice, rice syrup, and honey, the amount of overall sugars available in the product can be quite significant, even if the sugars may not be listed close to the top of the label. This is why looking at both the nutrition facts and the ingredients is so important.

Federal regulations do not prohibit a manufacturer from replacing the natural ingredients with chemical analogs, or substitutes. This means that the niacin, iron, vitamin B_1, B_2, and folic acid, which are all stripped from wheat products during processing, may be replaced with nutrients that are chemical in nature instead of from natural sources.

You can understand now that enriched products are not as healthy as whole foods. When you purchase whole grain pasta instead of enriched wheat pasta, you are buying a product that presents nutrients in a natural state. So you want to read that label to learn if "whole grain" is listed high on the list.

Any food that has been broken down is not a good choice. Further down in the ingredients we find milk protein concentrate (MPC); this is not the same as milk. Unfortunately we often don't read the entire label but focus on the words we know, leading many of us to think of this as milk. In reality MPC is a manufactured concentrated product often made by an ultrafiltration process, which reduces liquid milk to a powder, removing minerals and other substances while retaining 40 percent or more of the protein. It can also be found in products such as protein bars, yogurts, and frozen desserts. In addition to being a "fractionated" food, according to Food and Water Watch, a non-profit public interest group working to advocate and educate on the issues of clean food (including fish) and water, most of the MPCs in our food are imported from other countries and are not inspected for purity and safety.

Fractionated foods are foods that have been broken down with only part of that original food remaining in the processed item.

This makes MPC an ingredient you may not want to include in your pantry.

To understand packaged foods you cannot underestimate the importance of being aware of the ingredients on the label. If you do not know what an ingredient is, if you do not know how to pronounce it, or it is clearly chemical in nature (such as dyes, preservatives, and modified products) it is a safe bet that it is probably not food. We'll discuss different ingredients and their effects on your health in upcoming chapters.

FRONT OF PACKAGE CLAIMS

Often manufacturers will use the front of the box to make claims about their food. Part of the reason for doing this is to get consumers to bypass reading the nutrition label. Many people are confused about the label and choose instead to trust what it says on the front of the box. Unfortunately a number of claims that can be found on the front of a package can be misleading.

Let's start with the defined claims. These are claims that manufacturers make about their food for which the FDA has set certain standards.

1. **Free** — in order for a food to be marketed this way, such as "fat free" or "sugar free," it must have the least possible amount of the nutrient it is referring to. For example a fat-free food would need to provide less than .5 grams of fat per serving.

2. **Low** — foods that are marketed this way have slightly more of the nutrient than would be allowable for a "free" label. For example, a "low-fat" food would provide 3 grams or less of fat per serving. For cholesterol this number would need to be less than 2 grams per serving of saturated fat, while sodium would need to be 140 milligrams or less per serving.

3. **Reduced** — to qualify as a reduced food that item must have 25 percent less of that specific nutrient than the regular version of the same product. "Reduced fat" is a very common use of this claim.

All of these claims are based on serving size, not portion size. These serving sizes are often set by the manufacturers. Claims for which there are no regulations are the most confusing ones. Manufacturers know that consumers often key in to certain words or phrases — "low fat" or "sugar free." So they may take advantage of that and prominently display them on the front of the package.

These prominently displayed desirable characteristics, however, don't tell the full story. One prime example is the trend for whole grains. It can be very misleading to look at a loaf of bread and see "6 GRAINS" in bold, prominent print on the front of the package. While there may be 6 different grains in the bread, that statement is no guarantee that they are whole grains and certainly no guarantee that the first ingredient is a whole grain.

Whole grain products consist of all three parts of the plant's kernel: the bran, the inner endosperm, and the germ. Misleading information is also true with loaves that are marketed as "100% whole wheat." Whole wheat is not the same thing as whole grain, and manufacturers are counting on the fact that you don't know that. Whole wheat flour may have much of the germ removed. Therefore, 100% whole wheat bread may not be whole grain. Frequently whole wheat breads are made with enriched wheat flour as the first ingredient. You still need to flip that item over to look at the nutrition label.

Another silly example I see at the grocery store all the time applies to eggs. Many manufacturers proudly display "vegetarian fed hens" on their egg carton. Obviously someone decided that sounded good and it would be tempting to consumers. The problem with this statement is that chickens are not, by nature, vegetarians. While they do eat grains, vegetables, and fruits, they also like to eat bugs, worms, and moths, all of which provide protein and in exchange help create a healthier egg.

More startling than the misleading claims above are those that appear to make a health claim. Marketing cholesterol-free potato chips is nothing more than a way to try to convince you to buy a product that never had cholesterol in the first place.

Cholesterol comes primarily from animal fats and is found in items such as meats, eggs, and dairy.

Marketing ploys that appear to promote health add to the confusion. Claiming a cereal is high in healthy antioxidants and immune boosting nutrients is all well and good, but if it also comes laden with sugar, which is known to suppress the immune system, it's not a very valid or useful claim. [Baba. 1979] Rather than being swayed by manufacturing claims, it is important that you understand what you are really purchasing.

While this all sounds very confusing the good news is that you are in control. With the knowledge gained from this book you will become an informed consumer. This will give you the power to make conscious, healthy decisions that can have a positive effect for you and for your family.

YOUR LABEL READING ACTION PLAN

- Read the label.
- Calculate per serving — not per portion.
- Be aware of the sugars.
- Be aware of the fat content.
- If you do not understand an ingredient, don't eat it.

CHAPTER THREE

Understanding Additives

While food made at home from fresh ingredients is always tastiest and healthiest when it is eaten shortly after preparation, there has always been a need to prepare and process food. Traditionally, such techniques involved pickling, salting, fermenting, and smoking to meet the problems of safely storing food and avoiding food-borne illnesses. Most people do not have the time or the desire to preserve bacon or set up a root cellar. And who churns butter anymore?

In the first half of the 20th century, the United States was largely an agrarian society. Food tended to be locally grown and consumed. After World War II, more Americans began living in cities. Sophisticated food processing and preservation systems were developed to bring the food to the consumers. Such food processing methods required the inclusion of additives that would assure a wide range of safe, appealing, and convenient foods.

Today, food is produced on a large scale and delivered to local markets and shops. It must be transported and stored for some time before it reaches your pantry. And when you buy it you expect it to be healthful and of high quality. For most people this means they rely on the modern food industry to provide us with food that can be stored for some time and remain safe to eat.

Food additives make processed and convenience food possible. Your pantry is most likely stocked with products that you can prepare quickly and when you like, without worrying about daily shopping or spoilage. Additives are used for a number of reasons, including to maintain product consistency; to assure some nutritional value, especially if nutrients have been processed out; to prevent spoilage and contamination; and to enhance the flavor and color you expect to see in food. In short, additives enable food manufacturers to offer us products we would actually want to eat.

The food industry uses additives to assure a palatable texture, improve or preserve the nutrient value, reduce spoilage, improve the appearance, and enhance the flavor of our food. Additives keep the oil and water blended in that bottle of salad dressing. They keep your cereal from getting too soggy too soon. They keep gravy smooth and thick. And they make sure those Twinkies last six months—or six years —in the pantry without spoiling.

Today, authorities with the FDA carefully regulate food additives. Generally, the FDA requires approval of an additive before it can be used in food, and the manufacturer must prove that it is safe for the ways it will be used. So most people assume that if a substance is added to food, it must be safe. But is it healthful? Is it actually good for you?

Additives may be natural or man-made. Scientists are able to mimic natural flavors, color foods to make them look more natural, and preserve them for extended shelf life. Some foods are made entirely from chemicals, like coffee creamers and sugar substitutes.

Really, you ask? Food can be made entirely from chemicals? Yes. While government agencies like the US FDA supervise and regulate the use of additives in food, you don't necessarily want them in your pantry.

The term *additives* covers a very broad category of ingredients. Some of them are easy to identify; some of them are not quite as easy. This is also an area where people can quickly get very overwhelmed simply because there is so much to learn. As I've suggested before, pick one thing at time. Work on that, and when you have mastered it move on to the next item. Over time you will be surprised to see how many changes you have implemented that are now habits, easy to incorporate and not difficult to achieve. It all happens one step at a time.

TOP THREE NON-FOOD ITEMS

While there are many things —and I call them things because they are not food—that should not be part of your pantry, there are three that deserve special attention and that need to be removed from your pantry. They are high fructose corn syrup (HFCS), monosodium glutamate (MSG), and artificial colors. As I mentioned in the Introduction, there are a lot more than three things that don't belong in your pantry, but these are three really important ones. While the information relating to how they can affect your health can be startling, the important thing to remember is that you are in control. In this chapter you will learn why you don't want to eat these things; you'll also learn how to identify them so you can keep them out of your pantry and out of your meals. In this chapter I'll deal with HFCS, MSG, and other additives. You will find the information about artificial colors in Chapter Four.

HIGH FRUCTOSE CORN SYRUP

High fructose corn syrup is a sweetener that is very cheap. This makes it attractive to manufacturers. Part of the reason it's so cheap is due to governmental subsidies on corn and import taxes on foreign sugar. By reducing their sweetener costs, manufacturers can increase profits. There is, however, a growing backlash against HFCS. While producers claim that it is not unhealthy and have put together large ad campaigns to convince people to continue to use it, there is growing evidence to support its ill effects on our bodies.

Believed to contribute to obesity, diabetes, metabolic syndrome, and other diseases, HFCS is now undergoing more scrutiny. A Princeton University study from February 2010 clearly showed that rats that ate HFCS gained a lot more weight than those that ate table sugar, even though the two groups consumed the same number of overall calories. [Parker, 2010] This study should serve as a cautionary reminder that not all sweeteners, indeed not all calories, are created equal. Another study, published in 2009 in the journal *Obesity*, looked at the connection between non-alcoholic fatty liver disease (NAFLD), a condition generally linked to obesity and insulin resistance, and HFCS. NAFLD is essentially cirrhosis of the liver in people who don't drink alcohol, in other words a very dangerous health condition. [Collison, et al, 2009] The following year, in February 2010, another medical journal, *Practical Gastroenterology*, listed avoiding foods with HFCS as one of their top ten recommendations. Given these health concerns, HFCS is definitely an ingredient that does not belong in your pantry.

Just avoiding foods labeled with the name "high fructose corn syrup" may not be enough to keep it out of your pantry and your diet. When more and more consumers objected to the use of HFCS in their food, the Corn Refiners Association began to lobby to change the name to "corn sugars" in the hopes that a different name would make their product more appealing. [NYT. 2010] This petition was denied by the FDA, which stated the *"petition does not provide sufficient grounds for the agency to authorize 'corn sugar' as an alternate common or usual name for HFCS."* Unfortunately, however, there are other names under which HFCS hides when it comes to us in products from different countries. In Great Britain it is referred to as glucose-fructose syrup, while in Canada is it marketed as glucose/fructose. In Europe HFCS is sometimes referred to as isoglucose. Another hidden source is an ingredient called crystalline fructose. Made predominantly from corn with a fructose level of 98 percent, this powdered form is considered to be even sweeter than HFCS (and is often used as a substitute for HFCS in products such as frozen yogurt and various beverages). All of these forms are merely different names for a product that should be avoided.

While by no means a comprehensive list, here are a few commonly found items from the grocery store that contain HFCS*:

Capri Sun Juice Drinks
Coca Cola
Cool Whip
Dannon Fruit on the Bottom yogurts
Eggo Pancakes
Heinz Ketchup
Kellogg's Pop Tarts
Kraft Cheez Nips
Many Kellogg's cereals including Frosted Flakes, Corn Flakes,
    Raisin Bran, Special K, and Smart Start
Miracle Whip
Nabisco Fig Newtons
Nabisco Wheat Thins
Nutri-grain Bars
Planter's Trail Mix
Seagram's Tonic Water

Smuckers Uncrustables Peanut Butter/Strawberry Jam Sandwiches
Stovetop Stuffing
Yoplait Yogurts

*THIS LIST IS CORRECT AS OF DECEMBER 2012

In a surprising twist, HFCS can also appear in non-food consumables, specifically cigarettes. HFCS is added is to make the cigarettes taste sweeter, along with the other addictive and harmful chemical ingredients. Cigarette manufacturers are required to post the ingredients of their cigarettes online. A brief review of an RJ Reynolds ingredients list includes a maximum level of 4.49% HFCS in any brand of cigarette that they manufacture. If you need one, this is another good reason to stop smoking. [RJRT. 2010]

MONOSODIUM GLUTAMATE

Monosodium glutamate (MSG) is a sodium salt, sometimes referred to as free glutamic acid, which is used primarily as a flavor enhancer. It used to appear quite heavily in Chinese food, giving rise to what was called "Chinese restaurant syndrome." Some people appear to be very sensitive to the presence of MSG in their food and experience various illnesses ranging from headaches and flushing or sweating to numbness, tingling or burning on the face or neck, heart palpitations, chest pain, nausea, and weakness. [Mayo Clinic. 2010] It appears that these symptoms are not the only negative effects that MSG can have on our bodies. Discovering that it promotes inflammation of the liver, one study from 2008 concluded that MSG should be reviewed for safety and possibly removed from use. [Nakanishi, et al, 2008] Dr. Russell Blaylock, author of *Excitotoxins: The Taste That Kills*, classes MSG as an excitotoxin, a glutamate or other similar molecule that can damage or kill nerve cells by over-stimulating them. According to Dr. Blaylock, infant animals exposed to MSG have developed neurobiological problems even when that exposure was simply because their mothers were fed MSG in gestation. Pointing out that these developing brains can be four times more susceptible to excitotoxins, Dr. Blaylock feels that the exposure and subsequent change in brain function can be similar to human ADD and ADHD. [Blaylock, 2000]

Unfortunately MSG is not always easy to identify. Frequently found in salad dressings, sauces, flavored potato chips, seasoning mixes, and other highly processed foods, it can be one of the more difficult additives to remove from your pantry because it hides under dozens of different names.

The following list contains those ingredients that *always* contain MSG and definitely should be avoided. The "E" numbers refer to the European way of identifying additives, something important to know as more and more foodstuffs are imported from abroad.

Glutamic acid (E 620)
Anything "Glutamate" (E 621, E 622, E 623, E 624, E 625)
Anything "Hydrolyzed"
Anything "Autolyzed"
Yeast extract
Calcium caseinate, Sodium caseinate
Gelatin
Textured protein
"Soy Protein" anything

Below is another list of ingredients; these *frequently* contain MSG, or free glutamic acid. This list is a little more difficult to balance in your pantry as the processing may be done in a way that does not free up the glutamic acid. The decision to eat foods that contain these ingredients may require some research on your part.

Carageenan (E 407)
Bouillon, broth, stock
Anything "Flavors" or "Flavoring"
Maltodextrin
Citric Acid, Citrate (E 330)
Anything "Ultra-pasteurized"
Barley malt
Pectin (E 440)
Anything containing "enzymes"
Anything "fermented" (excluding traditionally fermented foods such as sauerkraut, kimchi, and kefir)

Anything "protein fortified"

Malt extract

Many forms of "whey" protein

Soy sauce

Seasonings

Remember, if you purchase something and then realize it has an unwanted ingredient in it, I strongly encourage you to return it to the grocery store. The grocery stores want your business, and you do not want these ingredients in your pantry.

ADDITIVES ARE NOT FOOD

Other "things" that appear in our food are a variety of different additives. Some are preservative chemicals added to foods essentially to keep them shelf stable, increasing the amount of time that they may be available for sale. Other types of additives that appear in food items include emulsifiers, which keep oils and water together in foods such as mayonnaise; stabilizers, which keep foods together during transport or storage; and flavorings. Artificial colors and sweeteners are two different types of additives that will be dealt with in future chapters. Not all additives are bad; there are natural additives such as vinegar used as a preservative or honey as an emulsifier. However, this selection deals with those additives that do not belong in your pantry.

Flavorings are often used to boost the flavor of a product or to give it a flavor that will trick our taste buds into thinking it is something it really isn't. According to the Code of Federal Regulations "flavoring can be defined as the essential oil, oleoresin, essence or extractive, protein hydrolysate, distillate, or any product of roasting, heating or enzymolysis, which contains the flavoring constituents derived from a spice, fruit or fruit juice, vegetable or vegetable juice, edible yeast, herb, bark, bud, root, leaf or similar plant material, meat, seafood, poultry, eggs, dairy products, or fermentation products thereof, whose significant function in food *is flavoring rather than nutritional.*" (emphasis mine) [21CFR101.22]

One flavoring item of especial concern is diacetyl, the chemical used to create the "buttery" flavor in microwaveable popcorn. It has been linked to lung disease in factory workers exposed to the vapors. In 2004 a lawsuit awarded $20 million to a factory worker for lung damage caused by working with diacetyl. "Microwave Popcorn Lung," or bronchiolitis obliterans syndrome, is not limited to factory workers. In September 2012 a Colorado man was awarded more than $7 million in damages; he developed the condition after consuming two bags of microwaveable popcorn a day for ten years. [Jaslow. 2012] While this excessive level of consumption is not likely to be repeated in a majority of households, these cases show that there can be a danger to consumers as well.

Diacetyl is so toxic that the United States Department of Labor issued a notice, the Hazard Communication Guidance For Diacetyl And Food Flavorings Containing Diacetyl, which states "Significant new information regarding the health effects of diacetyl and food flavorings containing diacetyl (FFCD) affects the information that must be conveyed to employers and employees under the Occupational Safety and Health Administration's (OSHA) Hazard Communication standard." [OSHA. 2012]

A new study published in *Chemical Research in Toxicology* shows that diacetyl can cause an accumulation of amyloid-β, which is positively linked with Alzheimer's disease. [More, et al. 2012] Because the fumes from the coating infuse the food and the steam released when you open the bag, it is difficult to avoid ingesting the substance. It can also be found in margarine (which would otherwise have no taste), shortenings, oils, food sprays, and candies, among other substances.

Thanks to recent legal judgments, diacetyl may be disappearing from most microwaveable popcorn from major brands, but you still want to check the label (which may just say "butter flavor"). Better yet, make own hot air-popped popcorn to preserve not only your health, but also potentially your memory.

As mentioned above, "natural flavor" on a label can be a code word for MSG. It can also be a way to hide ingredients that are considered natural, but when you know what they really are you might not choose to eat them. One such "natural flavor" is a substance called castoreum. Made from the anal gland secretions of beavers, it is most often used in those foods and beverages that are flavored vanilla, raspberry, or strawberry. While not highly utilized in the food industry, it is nonetheless used in food and its use is hidden by the generic term "natural." For those who smoke (and I urge you to quit) it can also be used to flavor cigarettes. Perhaps, hopefully, the thought of smoking beaver butt will encourage you to stop. [Burdock. 2005] [Di Justo. 2008]

Because "natural flavors" are listed exactly that way on the label, it can make it difficult to truly know what is being added to your food. The best option is to avoid their use altogether.

Preservatives are used to prevent the growth of mold and bacteria, to keep food from decomposing, or stop the ripening process until such time as it is convenient for the producer to deliver it to your grocery store. Many of these fall into the seven simple rules listed in Chapter One. Alphabet items include BHA, BHT, EDTA, and TBHQ. These stand for Butylated Hydroxyanisole, Butylated Hydroxytoluene, Ethylenediamine Tetraacetic Acid, and Tertiary Butylhydroquinone. Even when spelled out they are less than appealing. Other preservatives include items such as benzoates, propionates, nitrates, and sulfites. Many preservatives have the capacity to increase the symptoms of allergies, asthma, eczema, migraines, or digestive distress. [Papazian, 2006] Some of them can cause cancer or be otherwise toxic. [Hord, et al. 2009] [Winter, 2009] Traditional methods of food preservation such as freezing, smoking, or salting generally do not utilize these more toxic preservatives. Canning and pickling often utilize sugar, salt, or vinegar as a preservative. If you are canning or pickling products at home, or if you purchase foods that are created via these more traditional methods, it is a good idea to look at the ingredients and make sure they are not chemical in nature.

Emulsifiers keep foods from separating (think oil and water). Many possess anti-caking or anti-foaming properties and are used in whipped goods, while others control the rate of crystallization in foods such as peanut butter or shortenings. Emulsifiers such as eggs, honey, or mustard work quite well for binding together foods such as baked goods or sauces. However, the commercial emulsifiers, frequently found in creamy foods, soft drinks, frozen foods, many breads or baked goods, and spreads such as margarine, again fall under the Seven Simple Rules listed in Chapter One: capital letters, numbers, and unknown words.

Ill health effects for the following emulsifiers have mostly been observed through animal studies. Considering that we share up to 99 percent of our genes with mice, animal studies are generally recognized as valid for similar effects on humans. [Walton. 2002] One common emulsifier, carageenan, made from red seaweed, needs to be avoided in the diet. Not only due to the potential for free glutamic acid, or MSG, but also because of it's highly inflammatory effects on the gastrointestinal tract. Causing ulcerative colitis-like symptoms in laboratory animals and linked to colon cancer, carageenan is, sadly, allowed in organic foods in spite of it's negative health effects. [Cornucopia. 2012] Polysorbate 80, another common emulsifier, has been shown to have carcinogenic activity; in other words, it could cause cancer. [Bernard, et al. 2010][National Toxicology Program. 1992]

Other emulsifiers, such as propylene glycol, have an alternative use in antifreeze, and animal studies going back decades have shown that it can bring about depression of the central nervous system in animals. [Miller, et al, 1981] It also can be a cause of allergies and asthma in children or cause other skin problems. In the case of propylene glycol, it unfortunately may not always appear on the label, making it a very difficult ingredient to identify. Apparently it is covered under an FDA regulation covering "incidental food additive labeling," which allows the manufacturer to skip any mention of it on the label. [Choi, et al. 2010] [Cantazaro and Smith, Jr. 1991] [FDA. 2011] Propylene glycol is typically found in a wide variety of foods such as ice creams, yogurts, cakes and other sweets, beer, salad dressings, and in pre-made cookie and cake mixes. Because it does not always appear on the label, these may be foods you eventually want to make yourself in order to avoid consuming it.

Stabilizers are used to thicken foods and further increase the effect of emulsifiers, helping to prevent ingredients from separating. Stabilizers are frequently used to make food colors brighter and more consistent. They tend to be found in dressings, condiments such as mayonnaise, low-fat dairy products, and spreads such as margarine. Unfortunately there are also health risks posed by the use of stabilizers. One in particular, alginic acid, is odorless and tasteless but appears in many foods, especially ice creams and other frozen confections. In a study with rats it was shown to cause distention of the lower intestine, a bumpy bladder, and renal pelvic calcium deposits. Another, glycerol, is used as a plasticizer for the edible coatings that surround some meats and cheeses. It can irritate the mouth, lips, and other mucous membranes. [Winter, 2009] Other stabilizers include gelatin, which is rendered from bones and other animal parts, and pectin, created from fruit, both of which, as referenced above, may be a potential source of MSG.

Many people find themselves increasingly sensitive to chemical additives. That sensitivity, combined with the various health issues, makes a strong case for removing them from your pantry. Sue Dengate runs the Food Intolerance Network. A champion of the additive-free lifestyle, she highly recommends avoiding all artificial ingredients to be healthy and has created the handy reference sheet shown for you to use. The more you can avoid these ingredients in your pantry, the healthier you and your diet will be.

Avoid these additives

from www.fedup.com.au

COLOURS
102,104,110,122,123,124,127,129,
132,133,142,143, 151,155
natural colour 160b (annatto)

PRESERVATIVES

Sorbates	200, 201, 202, 203
Benzoates	210, 211, 212, 213
Sulphites	220, 221, 222, 223, 224, 225, 226, 227, 228
Nitrates, nitrites	249, 250, 251, 252
Propionates	280, 281, 282, 283

SYNTHETIC ANTIOXIDANTS

Gallates	310, 311, 312
TBHQ, BHA, BHT	319, 320, 321

FLAVOUR ENHANCERS

Glutamates incl MSG	620, 621, 622, 623 624, 625
Ribonucleotides	627, 631, 635
Hydrolysed Vegetable Protein (HVP)	

ARTIFICIAL FLAVOURS
No numbers since they are trade secrets

The table below highlights some foods that contain these additives:

ADDITIVE	CAN BE FOUND IN
Sorbate	Cooked fish, yogurt, sour cream, fudge, cottage cheese, margarine, mayonnaise, fruit juices, canned fruit, frozen fruit, pie fillings, jams, jellies, many dried fruits
Benzoate	Soda, lemonade, energy drinks, cider, margarine, fruit juices, pickles
Sulfite	Alcoholic beverages, pickles, olives, salad dressing mixes, wine vinegar, white sugar, shrimp, lobster, scallops, gelatin, jams, jellies, shredded coconut, maraschino cherries, canned vegetables, dried soup mixes
Nitrite/Nitrate	Hot dogs, lunchmeat, bacon, ham, smoked fish, processed meat
Propionate	Baked goods, dried milk, condensed milk, flavored milk, flavored yogurt, canned fish, alcoholic beverages, sports drinks, diet foods, vinegar, mustard
Gallate	Fats, oils, mayonnaise, shortening, baked goods, candy, dried meat, dried milk

It is important to remember that you are in charge of the contents of your pantry. While the information above may seem overwhelming at first, cleaning up your pantry can be done. Remember, this book is meant to be a reference, a guide for you to use as you move forward on your journey toward health. By choosing one item to modify at a time and utilizing the resources provided in this book, you will find that, step by step, you are making consistent, effective changes and creating your holistically healthy pantry.

NATURAL ADDITIVES

There are other additives appearing more frequently in foods on the grocery store shelves that are not necessarily harmful. Several of them are being used in the growing number of gluten-free products (which require extra binders and thickeners to make up for the loss of gluten in the flours), while others are in response to consumer demand for non-chemical additives. The following list is a quick run-down of some of these ingredients, intended to help you better understand them. Please note that any ingredient can cause a potential allergic reaction, so this list in no way indicates a complete lack of potential toxicity. However, these are natural additive substances that do not appear to have any significant health concerns attached to their use.

Acacia gum — made from the acacia tree; used to prevent crystallization of sugar and as a thickener for foods like jellies, gum, and candies.

Acetic Acid — found in a wide range of plants and fruits; similar to vinegar. Often used in cheeses, baked goods, condiments, and pickles.

Ascorbic Acid — a form of vitamin C; a preservative found in frozen fruits, dry milk, beer, juices, preserves, and cooked meat products.

Ascorbyl Palmitate — an ascorbic acid salt; prevents foods from going rancid and is also used to cure meats.

Agar Agar — made from seaweed; a substitute for gelatin.

Albumen — made from egg whites; an emulsifier. If you are allergic to eggs this additive should be avoided.

Astragalus Gummifier — also known as tragacanth; a gummy resin extracted from the astragalus plant. It is often used in modeling frosting as well as pharmaceutically in lozenges and pills.

Beta Glucan—obtained from either oats or barley, this soluble fiber is often found in baked goods as well as beverages or even some thickened dairy products.

Citric Acid—sometimes referred to as sodium citrate; made from fermenting the sugars in citrus fruit. It is used as a flavoring (it gives a tart flavor), as an acid-alkaline balancer, and for curing certain foods.

D-Alpha Tocopherol—made from vitamin E; a preservative that can keep oils from going rancid.

Guar Gum—made from guar beans; a stabilizer often found in frozen fruit, icings, and as a thickener for drinks. It's also a binding agent, which can be found in baked goods, dressings, and some dairy products.

Inulin—made from chicory, this produce can function as a binder, emulsifier, stabilizer, or texturizer.

Lactase—the enzyme that breaks down lactose (milk sugar).

Lecithin—made from eggs, soy, or corn, it is best to get this in its organic form, as there is a high probability that the soy and corn may be genetically modified. It is used as an emulsifier in chocolate, baked goods, frozen desserts, and vegetable and/or animal fat products. Lecithin is often used as an antioxidant in breakfast cereals and in sweets such as candy, chocolate, and baked goods.

Papain—derived from papaya; an enzyme that can be used to tenderize meat.

Pectin—available from the roots, stems, or fruits of certain plants, it is used as a thickener or stabilizer. Often found in jams, ice creams, and frozen desserts.

Soba—another name for buckwheat, often used in pasta products.

Sorghum—a grain that produces a very sweet syrup often used as a texturizer and/or sweetener.

Xanthan Gum — also called corn sugar gum, it is best to look for this in its organic form as otherwise the potential exists for it to come from GMO corn. Used as a thickener emulsifier or stabilizer often in dairy products or dressings.

GMO stands for Genetically Modified Organism. Also referred to as GM or GE, this designation identifies foods that have had their genetic material forcibly changed in some way. One example: fish genes were added to tomatoes so the antifreeze proteins in polar fish would protect the tomatoes from freezing. [Hightower, et al. 1991] This product launched consumer resistance against GMOs. While it was never brought to market commercially, other products have been developed, and there is a continuing debate about the feasibility and safety of GMO crops.

YOUR ADDITIVE ACTION PLAN

- Read the label.
- Learn which products are most likely to contain additives and look for other options or make them yourself.
- If you are a smoker, quit.

CHAPTER FOUR

Your Colorful Diet

We are inundated by messages to eat a colorful diet, to eat the colors of the rainbow. And it is good advice, if that rainbow comprises a wide variety of whole, seasonal foods such as apples, berries, winter or summer squashes, yams, dark leafy greens, eggplants, and more. Sadly we are also inundated by a rainbow of artificially colored foods: strawberry milk (which has no strawberries in it), cereal bars, yogurt, drink pouches, and the like.

You may ask why manufacturers use artificial colors. Often is it to improve the appearance of food, to hide seasonal variations in certain products, or to boost the color of products picked before they are ripe and truly ready to eat. They are also used to give a bright appearance to processed foods.

Color influences our perception of taste and fires neurons in the hypothalamus. It primes our minds to expect a certain flavor. Take, for instance, Cheetos. In one taste test, people were asked to evaluate a batch made without the artificial yellow coloring that turns the snack—and our fingers—orange. Their brains did not register much cheese flavor from the crunchy gray snack, even though nothing had been done to change the product except to leave out the food coloring.

Sometimes color will tell the brain to override our taste buds. When yellow coloring was added to vanilla pudding, tasters thought they were eating banana or lemon pudding.

We are, in a sense, hardwired to identify healthful foods by color, drawn to the yellow in lemons and butter, the red of apples and raspberries, the green of spinach and kale. And with the exception of blueberries, which tend toward purple, the colors blue and black are appetite suppressants. Our primitive minds tend to register these colors in food as toxic or spoiled.

Color additives first may have appeared in our diets as early as 1500 BCE with the colors created from natural substances such as paprika, turmeric, and saffron. Today we still use many of those same substances in foods that are naturally colored. Natural colors in this country tend to be made from the following, depending on what color is desired: beets, carrots, turmeric, paprika, elderberry juice, spinach, blackberries, blueberries, cherries, or red cabbage. As you look at the list you'll realize these are all foods with colorants that stain (ever tried to get beet juice out of white pants?). While the color produced from these may not be as bright or as consistent as artificial colors, they are still the best, healthiest choice as they come from whole foods rather than from chemicals.

Today, artificial colors are a petroleum product. Yes, petroleum, as in related to gasoline. This is not a substance that provides any health benefits whatsoever. Petroleum-based colors, first created from bituminous coal, were discovered in 1856. Cheaper and easier to manufacture, these chemically created colors, which were more consistent, blended well with the food and often had no detectable flavor. [FDA. 2003] By the early 1900s eighty artificial colors had found their way into many foods and cosmetics. The Pure Food and Drugs Act of 1906 banned artificial colors that were "injurious to health." By 1938, only fifteen synthetic colors were legal. Since then, more have been banned. Orange #1 was banned after Halloween in 1950, when children became ill after consuming candy colored with it. In 1976, Red #2 was banned when it was found to cause intestinal tumors in rats.

While it may sound good to have a certification process, this only means that there is at least a minimum amount of the specified color and no more than a certain maximum of contaminants or impurities. Unfortunately, legally acceptable contaminants can include substances such as lead, mercury, arsenic, and more. [Feingold Association. 2010] And while these artificial colors are tested to meet chemical standards, they are not tested for allergenic or other health issues.

In the last decade, overall colorant use has increased dramatically. From 2001 to 2011 Total Certified Color (meaning color batches that passed FDA testing and were approved for use in food, drugs, and cosmetics) rose from three million pounds to more than five million pounds — an increase of more than two million pounds of artificial color. [FDA. 2001 and 2011] Strangely, this number is at odds with other sources. According to the Feingold Association, in 2005 Americans consumed almost eighteen million pounds of artificial color. [Feingold. 2005] Whatever the number, the use of artificial colors in our food supply is growing. Moreover, this increase of petrochemical dyes in the food chain creates a growing, heavy toxic food burden on both children and adults.

The following table shows the increase of artificial colors in the diet over the last seventy years.

WHAT THE CHILD GROWING UP IN THE US IN THE 1940s GOT:	WHAT THE CHILD GROWING UP IN THE US TODAY GETS:
White toothpaste	Multi-colored toothpaste (sparkles)
Oatmeal	Instant oatmeal (turns milk blue)
Corn flakes	Fruity Pebbles
Toast and butter, jam	Pop Tarts
Whipped cream	Cool Whip
No vitamins (perhaps cod liver oil)	Brightly colored bubble-gum flavored chewables
Sample school lunch: Meatloaf, freshly made mashed potatoes, vegetable, milk, cupcake made from scratch	Sample school lunch: Highly processed foods loaded with synthetic additives, no vegetables, chocolate milk with artificial flavor
Sample school beverage: Water	Sample school beverage: Soft drink with artificial color, flavor, caffeine, and sweetener

TABLE USED WITH PERMISSION FROM DR. TIFFANY JACKSON

BY THE NUMBERS

Artificial colors in this country typically are identified by the color name and a number. The most common are Red #40, Yellow #5, and Yellow #6, which are responsible for almost 90 percent of the dyes used. These three dyes contain a substance called benzidene, a known carcinogen. This certainly makes for a valid argument against them and is a good reason to avoid them. [Potera. 2010] Others dyes currently in use are Blue #1, Blue #2, Green #3, Red #3. Then there are limited-use dyes. One is Citrus Red #2, which is known to cause chromosomal damage and has been shown to be carcinogenic to animals in high doses. Oranges are dipped in Citrus Red #2 so they will have the appearance of uniform color. The supposition is that since we do not eat the orange peels we will not be affected. [ToxNet. 2003] The other limited-use colorant is Orange B, which is limited strictly to use in hot dogs and sausage casings.

One artificial color that deserves particular attention here is caramel. Often perceived as a natural substance, caramel is actually a blend of ammonia and sulfites mixed with sugar. Another type of caramel color, made using only ammonia, appears in beer, soy sauce, balsamic vinegar, and other dark brown foods. [CSPI. 2011] In February 2011, the Center for Science in the Public Interest, a consumer advocacy group, urged the FDA to ban caramel coloring, citing studies showing that it could lead to lung, liver, or thyroid cancer. Given the amount of caramel coloring used in the United States in soft drinks alone, this could represent a potentially significant carcinogenic exposure. Obviously as we look around us at the wide range of caramel-colored foods and soft drinks, this ban has not happened.

Many products manufactured in this country using artificial colors are produced without those artificial colors when sold in other countries. Kraft, Kellogg, McDonald's, Mars, PepsiCo, and other companies all make their products with natural colorings for the overseas markets where they have either been outlawed or legislation now requires a warning label. [CSPI. 2010] Instead of removing these artificial colors from their products altogether, the manufacturers have quietly continued to make those products for the US market. While it would seem to make sense to remove artificial colors from all versions of the product, because these chemical colors are allowed in the United States and because they are cheaper manufacturers continue to use them.

In March 2011 the FDA heard arguments about whether or not artificial colors at least should be labeled in this country. Sadly, in spite of the case presented to them, the panel voted against requiring a warning label on foods that contain artificial colors. [BusinessWeek. 2011] We can only hope that this will be reviewed in the near future so that these chemical colorants will not only be labeled but even banned. There is no need whatsoever for artificial colors in food; the use of them is merely a matter of convenience and cost for the manufacturer. Fortunately for those who take the time to read the label, artificial colors are clearly identified and easy to avoid.

IT'S IN WHAT?

So where are all of these artificial colors hiding? Obviously everyone can guess at or identify those cereals and candies with artificial color without having to read the label. But you may be surprised at the overwhelming number of foods that hide petrochemicals. Have you ever considered products such as pickles? Manufacturers use artificial colors to stabilize the appearance of their pickles. We have been conditioned to accept the artificially enhanced color of certain foods as natural. Artificial colors can also be found in food products such as salad dressings, marshmallows, pie filling, jellies, and juices. When you read the labels you may be startled to realize exactly how much artificial color is in the foods you have been buying and consuming.

Artificial colors appear in a wide range of products such as vitamins, mouthwashes, medications, and cosmetics as well as food. If you eat, swallow, or wear artificial colors from these other sources, you are getting significant exposure to them. Yes, even wearing them can cause a problem. Remember that the skin is the largest body organ. What you put on it will make its way into your system. It's important to know that artificial colors are not always clearly identified on the label of non-food items; sometimes they are simply referred to as "colorant." However, just as with food, as you are wandering the aisles of the store purchasing a variety of products, read the label to find the colorants and you will be able to avoid them successfully.

ATTENTION DEFICIT DISORDER

In 2007 the BBC published a news article highlighting findings from the University of Southampton, a leading research-led university in Southampton, England, showing a link between artificial colors and temper tantrums, allergic reaction, and poor concentration in children. In the study, three hundred children were tested under a double-blind study with the artificial colors tartrazine, ponceau, sunset yellow, carmoisine, quinoline yellow, and allura red as well as the preservative sodium benzoate. The children tested belonged to two different age groups, three-year-olds and eight- to nine-year-olds. This research supported findings from a previous UK study done seven years earlier linking artificial colorants to allergic reactions and ADHD-type behaviors. The UK experts recommended parents stop giving their children these additives. [McCann. 2007]

While it is not clear if the chemical composition of the artificial colorings is exactly the same in the United States as in the United Kingdom, this study upheld the findings of Dr. Ben Feingold, a prominent pediatrician and allergist who was Chief of Allergy at the Kaiser Permanente Medical Center in San Francisco. In 1968 Dr. Feingold published "Recognition of Food Additives as a Cause of Symptoms of Allergy." Throughout his career he published many articles and worked in clinical practice encouraging families to remove additives from their diet. The Feingold Association, founded in 1976, continues to promote a diet that eliminates artificial ingredients, flavorings, colorants, and preservatives. Dr. Feingold claimed as many as 50 percent of his hyperactive patients showed an improvement in behaviors after colorants were removed from their diet. [CSPI. 1999]

ANNATTO AND COCHINEAL

Although some natural colors are made from metals such as iron or extracted using toxic solvents, the majority of those recommended for use are from vegetable or plant sources and are low on the allergenic scale. However, two natural color additives, annatto and cochineal, have high allergenic potential, making it important to be aware of their presence.

Annatto, also infrequently listed as bixin or bixaceae, is considered a natural color and therefore exempt from regulation. Created from tropical tree seeds, it is a vegetable dye that gives food an orange-yellow appearance. Commonly found in cheeses, crackers, cereals, and other food products, annatto also may be present when the ingredients list shows "artificial color" or "color added." Because it is considered a natural color it does not have to be specifically identified. This can present a problem, as there are increasing numbers of allergic or other health concerns linked to its use, including irritable bowel syndrome, urticartica, asthma, and other typical allergic reactions. [Food Intolerance Network. 2010]

Cochineal extract, another natural colorant, sometimes called carmine, is made from the crushed dried bodies of female Costa insects and appears in both food and cosmetics. It is used where a red color is needed and may be referred to as cochineal dye, carmine, carminic acid, or natural color. Examples of foods that could contain cochineal extract include yogurt, cranberry juice drinks, ice cream, and some candies. Vegetarians, of course, do not choose to consume it, as it is from an animal source.

In March 2012 CBS News reported that Starbucks had changed the recipe for their Strawberries and Cream Frappuccinos, adding cochineal extract for the color. The reaction from consumers was immediate and quickly went viral. Not only do vegetarians and vegans oppose the use of the bugs; it appears that many other consumers were upset at the thought of bugs in their drink and questioned their use. A Change.org petition was started. In very short order Starbucks responded to consumer demand and returned to using food-based sources for color.

Workers exposed to cochineal extract have reported incidents of asthma. Others have experienced dermal reactions to lip salve colored with cochineal extract and a wide variety of allergic reactions, including anaphylaxis, after eating or drinking substances containing cochineal. [Inchem. 2000] Because of the severity of these reactions the FDA implemented a rule which states, "*The Food and Drug Administration (FDA) is revising its requirements for cochineal extract and carmine by requiring their declaration by name on the label of all food and cosmetic products that contain these color additives. This final rule responds to reports of severe allergic reactions, including anaphylaxis, to cochineal extract-containing food and carmine-containing food and cosmetics and will allow consumers who are allergic to these color additives to identify and thus avoid products that contain these color additives.*" [FDA. 2009] This labeling represents a positive step in helping consumers to make informed decisions about purchasing products with these ingredients.

A number of manufacturers are starting to make changes, choosing to use natural food colors. Given the increasing health issues and the concerns about the negative effects of artificial colors in the food supply, your switch to natural foods colors is advisable. Food colorings can be created from readily available food sources such as beets for a red tint, spinach for a green tint, carotene (from carrots) for orange, or saffron for yellow. For homemade goods there are several sources of plant-based food dyes, which can be purchased in stores or on the Internet.

As a consumer it is important to read the labels on all food products to learn which products do not contain petrochemical dyes and thus be able to make the choice for a chemical-colorant-free diet. The wide range of products that have artificial colors in them is startling and disappointing. Although the colors from natural food sources are not as brilliant or as consistent as petrochemical dyes, an effort needs to be made toward avoiding the inherent health issues arising from consuming artificial food colors. We need to learn to change our perception of what represents acceptable color variations within our food supply. Additionally, manufacturers need to be further encouraged to remove artificial food colors from their products and to replace them with colorants from natural sources. A large part of this change, this encouragement, comes from consumers, people like you and me, making the choice to not purchase artificially colored products.

YOUR ARTIFICIAL COLOR ACTION PLAN

- Read the label so you can identify artificial colors.
- Remember artificial colors are made from coal tar and/or its derivatives; avoid them.
- Be aware that annatto and cochineal extract are natural food colorings that can cause allergies or other health issues.
- Also check personal care products, cosmetics, supplements, and medications for artificial colors.

CHAPTER FIVE

Trick or Treat? Understanding Sugars

Two hundred years ago, US consumption of added sugar was 6.3 pounds per person per year. Now it is more than one hundred pounds per person each year!

Do you find it hard to believe any single person could eat so much sugar? Consider: the average American eats approximately twenty-one teaspoons of added sugar a day. That's almost two and a half times the recommended amount of six teaspoons (just 24 grams) of added sugar per day for women and nine teaspoons (36 grams) per day for men. How much do you spoon into your morning coffee? (A sugar packet contains a teaspoon.) How much might be in that bowl of ice cream you enjoyed last night? Probably 28 grams per serving, or seven teaspoons. (And we've already talked about the likelihood of eating just one serving!) Okay, so maybe you drink your coffee black and never eat dessert. How about that small cup of low-fat, fruit-flavored yogurt? It likely had seven teaspoons of added sugar, *more* than the recommended amount for women.

"Added sugar" means sugar not found naturally in foods like fruits and milk. They are the sugars in processed and prepared foods such as desserts, sweets, cereals, soft drinks, fruit juices, sauces, and salad dressings. (A cup of orange juice has more than five teaspoons.)

According to the US Department of Agriculture (USDA) sugar is the most common food additive. We could call it "hidden sugar," because it's found in many foods that we do not normally think of as having it, such as lunchmeat, crackers, condiments, and soups. By adding sugars to these foods manufacturers influence our taste preferences so we expect things to taste sweeter than they might otherwise, without realizing how many extra calories we are consuming. A tablespoon of ketchup contains one teaspoon of sugar (more likely high fructose corn syrup).

Part of our sugar intake is manipulated by the glycemic index of the foods we eat. This term refers to a measure of how quickly our bodies break down our food, releasing glucose into our bloodstream. Simple carbohydrates, highly processed foods, and sugars all break down quickly. The more complex foods are digested more slowly and therefore have a lower impact on blood sugar. The glycemic index is represented by percentages with glucose being given a value of 100, which is the top of the scale. Eating lower on the glycemic index means less sugar in our systems. Values for glycemic index are broken down in the following way:

	GLYCEMIC INDEX	EXAMPLES
Low	Less than 55	Most fruits and vegetables, legumes, most whole grains, and nuts
Medium	55 to 69	Whole wheat products, rice, and potatoes
High	70 and above	White bread, extruded breakfast cereals, any crackers and cookies

Eating too many calories from sugar (glucose) or higher glycemic foods can have a negative impact on the metabolism. The body utilizes the sugar we eat by signaling the pancreas to produce insulin. The insulin in turn helps the sugar enter into our tissues. Insulin also signals the liver to store glycogen. The more sugar we take in, the more insulin our pancreas releases. High levels of insulin force the liver to store as much as it can for later. The body takes these "extra" calories and stores them as adipose, or fatty tissue. The more insulin there is, the slower the body responds to breaking down this fat. In very simple terms this can lead to weight gain. Repeated high exposure to sugar, and therefore insulin, can over time potentially lead to a blunted response to insulin, which is sometimes referred to as insulin resistance or metabolic syndrome. Further negative biological responses to this overabundance of sugars can include high blood pressure or a negative effect on cholesterol and triglycerides. In many cases continued insulin resistance can eventually lead to diabetes.

Eating too much sugar also has the potential to affect your hormones. One study from 2007 showed that eating too much sugar could turn off the gene that regulates active testosterone and estrogen. When the liver metabolizes excess sugar, whatever the body can't use right away is turned into lipids. Scientists found that this increased production of lipids shuts down the sex hormone binding globulin (SHBG) gene. This reduces the amount of SHBG protein in the blood. With reduced SHBG protein the levels of testosterone and estrogen rise. These higher levels of hormone have been associated with acne, infertility, and polycystic ovaries, among other illnesses. [Science Daily. 2007]

Combining the concern of hormone-related illness with a national increase in rates of diabetes and obesity, it is clear that we need to understand the different forms of sugar, including artificial sugars, and how to limit them in our pantries and our diets. Reading the label to see how many grams of sugar are listed in the nutrition facts is an important start. Also important is reading the ingredients list. Often manufacturers will use more than one kind of sweetener in a product to make it look like there is less sugar. Remember from Chapter Two: the higher up an ingredient is listed, the more of that ingredient there is in the product. If the manufacturer uses three or five different kinds of sweeteners, they can use less of each one, and those ingredients drop lower on the list. You'll need to look at both the amount of sugar and the kinds of sugar to get a true picture of just how much you may be consuming.

For the balance of this chapter I am going to focus on the various forms of sugar that are added to our diet. In this chapter we discuss sugars in three categories: complex, refined, and artificial. Learning about various sugars as sweeteners and what effects they can have on the body will inspire you to identify them at the grocery store. The goal is to gain an understanding of these different types of sugars and then, utilizing your label-reading skills, to limit your intake.

COMPLEX SUGARS

Quantity and the degree of refinement strongly influence the health impacts of various sugars. Complex, low-, and unprocessed sugars are slower to enter the bloodstream. It is important, however, to remember that even though a sugar may be more complex, it is still a sugar, it still provides calories, and it still should be limited. Those calories can be varied depending on what kind of sugar it is. Comparing two popular sweeteners used in drinks, an average level teaspoon of sugar weighs 4 grams and contains fifteen calories while a teaspoon of honey weighs 7 grams and contains twenty-one calories. This highlights the fact that not all sugars are equal and that they all can still represent a significant caloric density (a lot of calories for a small amount).

Complex sugars include brown rice syrup, barley malt syrup, whole fruit purees, fruit sauces, honey, maple syrup, date sugar (made from ground dried dates), agave nectar, coconut sugar (made from coconut palm blossoms), and molasses.

Also included in the complex sugars category are low-process sugars that include an unrefined cane juice sometimes referred to as Sucanat, which stands for SUgar CAne NATural. Sucanat is a dark, low-process sugar that retains much of it's mineral content giving a rich, complex flavor. Other lower process sugars include muscovado, a large crystalline, somewhat sticky sugar. Turbinado, sometimes referred to as raw sugar, makes a good substitution for brown sugar as it has a good moisture content. Demerara sugar is a lighter, more golden color than muscovado or turbinado with a larger, dry crystal structure making it a good choice for sprinkling on top of cookies, muffins or other baked goods.

Although it is a whole food, fruit is also a source of sugar; along with the fructose (fruit sugar) it contains fiber, vitamins, and minerals. While the fruit sugar, which is available in varying amounts depending on the fruit, will have an effect on your system, the fiber can moderate or slow down the body response especially in the harder, more fibrous fruits. However, when you consume sugar, any sugar from any source, your body responds. Remember, taking in too much sugar can have a negative effect on your metabolism.

Agave nectar is considered a complex sugar, however, it is primarily fructose. Reports place its fructose content at levels of up to 90 percent (higher than the 55 percent fructose of HFCS). [Mercola and Pearsall. 2006] Its primary attraction is that it has a low-glycemic index. However, as noted in Chapter Three, high fructose sweeteners are difficult for your liver to process and should be avoided. [Mercola. 2010]

Although current recommendations from the USDA call for five to nine servings of fruits and vegetables per day, that number is skewed. We should be eating far more vegetables than fruit each day.

Many people include stevia (Stevia rebaudiana) in the complex sugar category even though it is not a sugar per se. Stevia, a sweet herb from South America, has up to three hundred times the sweetness of white sugar, yet it does not cause a rise in blood sugar. It also has no calories, making it a sweetener of choice for those desiring to limit their sugar consumption. There is a limited subset of people for whom stevia has an unpleasant aftertaste. Often this can be mitigated by using mostly stevia with a very small amount of honey or other complex sweetener to mask the aftertaste. Some manufacturers have begun to make stevia in a form that is mixed with a modest amount of sugar. This mixture does supply a few calories; however, it is far less than the amount provided in other forms of sugar, making it a low-calorie choice. Stevia is available in many grocery stores and comes in either a liquid or powder form.

REFINED SUGARS

The body more quickly utilizes refined, or simple, sugars because they are more highly processed. They are also stripped of minerals and other nutritional benefits. Examples of refined sugars include white sugar, brown sugar (this is typically white sugar with a light coating of molasses for color), high fructose corn syrup, inverted sugar syrup (often found in candies), and concentrated fruit juices. Many vegans (people who eat no animal product whatsoever) choose not to eat white sugar because it may be processed through a bone char filter.

Unfortunately many of the calories consumed from refined sugar are empty calories, found in soft drinks, candies, and other sugary substances. The term *empty calories* refers to those calories taken in that provide no nutritional benefit. When we eat empty calories our bodies still require fuel, so we may end up eating more to get the calories we need. However, we're also taking in the extra non-nutritional calories. Those extra calories get turned into fat, affecting the body negatively, as I've discussed.

SUGAR ALCOHOLS

The refined sugar category also includes sugar alcohols, which are not really sugar but are sweet. Made by adding hydrogen to sweet substances, the sugar alcohols are extracted. (The exception to this process is erythritol, which is made by fermentation.) They are a carbohydrate that is sweet but has around half of the calories of sugar. Sugar alcohols can be found in a wide range of products, especially dietetic ones, such as candies, baked goods, syrups, and ice creams. Sugar alcohols are usually identified by the -ol at the end of their name: erithritol, xylitol, lacitol, malitol, mannitol, polyglycitol, and sorbitol. One exception to the -ol rule is isomalt, which is another form of sugar alcohol. Since they are not completely digested when eaten, sugar alcohols can cause bloating and gas or have a laxative effect. Because they are "created" sweeteners, and due to the potential negative physical effect, sugar alcohols should be taken in moderation.

ARTIFICIAL SWEETENERS

A sugar substitute, or artificial sweetener, is an additive that tastes like sugar, but generally has few or no calories. High-intensity sweeteners are many times sweeter than sugar, so less is needed to get the same sweet taste. Some are derived from natural sources, but most are artificial, made from chemicals.

The first artificial sweetener ever created was saccharin. Discovered in 1879, it is a derivative of coal tar. Artificial sweeteners became very popular because of their low- or zero-calorie content, leading many to believe that they were preferable to natural sweeteners. Artificial sweeteners also allowed diabetics to eat sweet foods like cake and cookies, since there is no actual sugar present.

Current artificial sweeteners are: saccharin, aspartame (NutraSweet™ or Equal™), sucralose (Splenda™), neotame (another form of NutraSweet™), and acesulfame potassium (Sunett™ and SweetOne™). There are also two artificial sweeteners made with a chemical extract from stevia. I'll address those below.

As of this writing, two more artificial sweeteners are currently pending FDA approval, Alitame and Cyclamate (which was banned in 1970 and is currently seeking re-approval with the FDA).

Artificial sweeteners have been shown to have various adverse health effects. In the 1970s the USDA banned saccharine because studies revealed a risk for cancer of various organs including bladder, uterus, ovaries, and skin. In the late 1990s the Calorie Control Council argued that the studies finding bladder cancer in male rats did not correlate to a risk to humans. As a result the ban was overturned. This was despite the fact that animal studies are well respected as a means of identifying potential hazards with foods, medications, and other substances.

When it comes to animal testing of products to verify its safety in humans, the FDA requires at least two animal studies, one in rats and one in mice. This causes confusion for the consumer when manufacturers or the government are willing to accept the results of a particular animal study but then reject the results of a different study claiming it doesn't apply because it is "only" an animal study. We share approximately 99 percent of our genes with mice, and 80 percent of our genome has a one-to-one counterpart between each species. This flip-flop between acceptance and non-acceptance of studies appears to be more a matter of convenience for the manufacturer and a lack of compliance with standards rather than a firm way to measure effectiveness and safety.

Now aspartame has come under scrutiny with a recent study from a highly respected Italian cancer institute showing an increase in lymphomas, leukemias, and breast cancer in rats. As a result of this study the Center for Science in the Public Interest (CSPI) has downgraded aspartame, labeling it "everyone should avoid" instead of its previous "use caution" rating. [CSPINET. 2007] Of course, there is some controversy regarding this issue because the study was based on animal studies.

Splenda's Not So Sweet: Splenda, which is touted as being "from sugar," is another artificial sweetener that isn't all it's cracked up to be. This chemical creation became the first of what appears to be a new trend in artificial sweeteners: breaking apart and re-assembling whole ingredients to make a chemical counterpart that has reduced calories. While part of the ingredient list may indeed include a natural substance (in the case of Splenda, it's sugar), the product itself certainly is not natural.

The claim is that Splenda is made from sugar but has no calories. The reality isn't so benign. Splenda was discovered when a misunderstanding in a laboratory led to one of the laboratory assistants tasting (rather than "testing") an experimental chlorinated sugar that was being developed as an insecticide. This led to the realization that chlorinated sugars taste sweeter than sugar. [Mercola and Pearsall. 2006] But while chlorine combines readily with the sucrose molecule for sugar substitution, the chlorine itself must be chemically altered so that it doesn't break down inside the body. So neither the sugar nor the chlorine is in a natural state by the time this artificial sweetener is created. Far from it: chlorinated sugars are also in the same chemical class as perchloroethylene, a carcinogenic dry cleaning fluid, and the banned insecticides DDT and chlordane. And yet Splenda, essentially a chlorinated sugar, is classified by the FDA as GRAS (generally recognized as safe).

We may be doing more damage to our health than we know by ingesting Splenda. Some studies have indicated that the use of Splenda could create intestinal changes that limit the benefit of oral medications. [Abu-Donia, et al. 2008] A Duke University study found evidence that average-to-high consumption levels of Splenda reduced beneficial bacteria levels in the intestines of rats by as much as 50 percent. These beneficial bacteria are an important component of our intestinal flora and help to keep our gut healthy. They keep our digestion strong, improve nutrient absorption, support our immune system, and help promote healthy elimination. Reducing their levels might have a negative impact on intestinal function.

Although the manufacturers would like you to think that Splenda is "just like sugar," it's not.

Truvia's Not Too Terrific: Two of the newest stars on the artificial sweetener billboard are Truvia™ and PureVia™. Both of these new sweeteners, just like Splenda, are touted as being from "natural" substances, in this case stevia.

It is of concern among a number of scientists and nutrition professionals that, similar to the introduction of other artificial sweeteners, these substances have been approved too quickly. Sadly for the consumer, these concerns have been brushed aside in the rush to bring these products to market. Even sadder, history may be repeating itself. Aspartame and saccharin used to be the stars of the non-nutritive sweetener (fancy words for artificial sweetener) world. After they were approved as GRAS by the FDA (in spite of mounting evidence that they might not be safe for human consumption), it was eventually discovered that they were in fact harmful. Now we have new products on the shelf as manufacturers desperately try to profit from the American public's desire to consume fewer calories without actually eating less or making healthier choices.

The newest media and marketing darling, Truvia, born from a partnership between Coca-Cola and Cargill, apparently is created from an isolated extract from the stevia leaf called rebiana. The stevia herb grows primarily in South America, is related to the chrysanthemum, and is approximately 300 times sweeter than sugar. Stevia has been used in South America for centuries and is used in many countries around the world with no known ill effects. Studies in journals such as *Metabolism: Clinical and Experimental* and *Clinical Therapeutics* show the health benefits of stevia in its ability to improve insulin sensitivity in rats and the possibility of reversing diabetes and metabolic syndrome. [Chang, et al. 2005] However, those health benefits apply only to stevia, not to its chemical analogues.

Once disallowed for use in human consumption, until recently stevia was available for sale only as a dietary supplement, primarily in health food stores. In 1991 the FDA banned stevia, claiming that there was insufficient evidence to demonstrate its safety.

The FDA still hasn't approved the use of stevia as a food additive. Nevertheless, in a quiet reversal in December of 2008, the FDA issued a "no objection" approval to GRAS status for the use of stevia in Truvia. With that approval the rush to market this new sugar substitute began. Fortunately it brought with it mainstream access to stevia. However, many consumers are mislead by the advertising and believe that Truvia is the same as stevia, when in fact it isn't.

Because the artificial sweetener market is so profitable, other companies are determined to get a piece of the pie, creating competing products. PepsiCo has now created their version, which they call PureVia. These names are marketing genius, Truvia — true...meant to make you believe it is a true food product, PureVia — pure...meant to make you believe it's not a manufactured product, presumably meant to bring up imagery of a plant or a natural substance. And wading into the fray are the other artificial sweeteners, Zerose, Zevia, and Zsweet, which appear to be made from a base of stevia and erythritol.

These new artificial sweetening products are severely under-tested and might, in the future, prove to be detrimental to your health. Currently, Cargill has sponsored most of the studies available for Truvia. The CSPI reveals that studies done at the University of California Los Angeles (UCLA) show a concern among scientists that this creation has not been adequately tested. As mentioned above, the FDA typically requires animal studies in both rats and in mice before they will consider a product for approval. In spite of this requirement Truvia has as of this writing been tested in rats, with some concerning results. Additionally it has not been tested in mice. And yet, unfortunately it has been approved for use by people.

One scientist, Curtis Eckhert, professor of toxicology at UCLA, points out that this sweetener may wind up being consumed by tens of millions of people who will be exposed to it through soft drinks and other products. He is pushing for further studies before the products can be considered truly safe.

So while Cargill will now attempt to promote Truvia as a being "just like stevia" (as will PepsiCo for PureVia), don't be fooled. Truvia and PureVia are not "just like" stevia. Only stevia is stevia. These other sweeteners are created versions that are similar, but they are most definitely not the same.

OTHER HEALTH CONCERNS

Our willingness to consume artificial sweeteners may be doing us more harm than good. Research from Purdue University reveals that artificial sweeteners may confuse the ability of the body to "count" calories based on sweetness. This could reduce what should be a natural ability to regulate our caloric intake. [Davidson and Swithers. 2004] Further research has also indicated a positive relationship between the use of artificial sweeteners and weight gain. [Yang. 2010] Also of concern for many consumers, both sucralose and aspartame have been implicated in triggering migraines. [Bigal, et al. 2006] [Newman and Lipton. 2001] All of these are very good reasons to avoid artificial sweeteners, no matter what their source, and keep them out of your pantry.

YOUR SUGAR ACTION PLAN

- Learn what the various sugars are.
- Read the label to understand how many sugars are in your food; many products on the grocery store shelves can contain more than one type of sugar.
- Look for products that have sugar listed lower down in the ingredients list. If at all possible you do not want sugar to be listed in the first five ingredients.
- As we discussed in Chapter One, HFCS is one of the top three products to remove from your pantry. However, anything that falls under the Refined Sugar, Sugar Alcohol, or Artificial Sweeteners categories also should be removed.
- Limit your sugars; anything that falls under the Complex Sugar category is a reasonable choice but should be consumed only in moderation.
- Remember the six or nine teaspoon per day recommendation.
- Remember to consider sugars from all sources, including fruit and fruit juices.

CHAPTER SIX

The Skinny on Fats

Our relationship with healthy fats has been derailed. We are surrounded by messages telling us that fat is not good for us and we should be eating less of it. This is not true! Healthy fats are an important part of our diet. Fat is required to help with hormone production, to manage hunger symptoms, to process fat-soluble vitamins, and more. When we eat reasonable amounts of healthy fats, this helps to maintain a healthy body state. However not all fats are created equal.

In an attempt to tap into the health-conscious market many manufacturers make fat-free or low-fat products. These products are very unhealthy. The removal of fat also removes the flavor. To make up for this many of these products contain high levels of sugar, salt, and potential MSG ingredients. In a startling twist, it turns out that when we eat low-fat or no-fat foods, we often eat more, simply because we think it's "healthier." [Wansink. 2006]

Fats can be a confusing topic, as some foods contain multiple types of fat. To keep things simple, for the purposes of this chapter I will focus primarily on those fats used for cooking so you can choose those sources that are most supportive to your health. We'll start with an overview, defining different types of fat.

SATURATED FATS

Saturated fats are found primarily in animal products. The word *saturated* refers to the number of hydrogen bonds in the fatty acid chains. Because the fat molecule is fully saturated with hydrogen atoms, it cannot incorporate more. Animal products with saturated fat include dairy products such as cream, cheese, and butter. Other forms of saturated animal fats are suet, the hard fat found around the loins and kidneys in beef or mutton; tallow, the processed form of suet;

and lard, which is pig fat. Vegetable sources of saturated fats include coconut oil, cottonseed oil, and palm kernel oil.

It is important to remember that, contrary to popular misconception, saturated fats are not all bad. They are, in fact, biologically required as a basis for hormone production, organ padding, and energy metabolism.

One saturated fat in particular, coconut oil, has been vilified as an unhealthy fat. This myth arose when scientists first began to study fats and their effect on heart health. They used hydrogenated coconut oil, a form of trans-fat, in their studies. Coconut oil does not require hydrogenation. It may be solid at room temperature (if it's cold enough), is shelf stable without hydrogenation, and, furthermore, provides beneficial medium chain fatty acids.

As Bruce Fife, ND, writes in *The Healing Miracles of Coconut Oil*, until the 1980s, coconut oil was popular for baking, frying, and even making popcorn at movie theaters. In an effort to commandeer the market, domestic vegetable oil manufacturers, including the American Soybean Association, launched a battle to discredit imported tropical oils. Backed by nutrition experts who claimed that coconut oil was a saturated fat that caused heart disease, the American food industry prevailed over poorer developing countries exporting coconuts, and food manufacturers — and movie theaters — replaced coconut oil with partially hydrogenated soybean oil.

Coconut oil is innocent of the charges, and actually has many virtues. Rather than being the unhealthy fat we've all been led to believe it is, coconut oil appears to have a neutral effect on blood cholesterol levels and at the same time stimulate the metabolism. [Fife. 2004] Additionally, studies show that it can help reduce belly fat. [Assunção, et al. 2009]

MONOUNSATURATED FATS

Found in many foods considered part of the heart-healthy Mediterranean diet, monounsaturated fats (MUFA) can be found in olives, olive products, avocados, avocado oil, nuts, and seeds. They tend to be liquid at room temperature. These fats have been shown to reduce overall cholesterol levels while at the same time reducing LDL, or "bad," cholesterol. MUFAs have also been shown to help prevent accumulation of belly fat and may decrease insulin resistance, making it a positive choice for those with diabetes or metabolic resistance. [Paniagua, et al. 2007]

One MUFA source to watch out for, however, is canola oil. The word *canola* stands for CANadian Oil, Low Acid. The oil is made from rapeseed, a brassica related to turnips, cabbage, and Brussels sprouts. It is important to note that while canola is rich in MUFAs, contrary to popular belief it is not a healthy choice for the diet. Along with soy, canola is one of the most overwhelmingly contaminated GMO crops and therefore should be avoided. You can read more about GMO in Chapter Seven.

POLYUNSATURATED FATS

Although they can include omega-3 fatty acids, and we all know we need more of those in our diet, polyunsaturated fatty acids (PUFA) can be very unstable and prone to oxidization. Like MUFAs, PUFAs tend to be liquid at room temperature. Exposure to light, air, moisture, and especially heat can cause a reaction that subjects the body to high levels of free radicals, which may be linked to diseases such as cancer, heart disease, autoimmune dysfunction, and premature aging. [Enig and Fallon. 2005] PUFAs can be found in corn, safflower, soy, and canola oils as well as in some seeds and nuts.

FAKE FATS

Man-made or chemically created fats are not healthy choices as they can have significantly negative health effects.

Olestra, sometimes called Olean, was approved for use in food the mid-1990s and initially intended for use in high fat prepared foods such as potato chips. Because it is not easily digested, olestra effectively lowers the fat content by passing virtually unchanged through the digestive system. Unfortunately, consumption of olestra was often accompanied by loose, watery stools, "anal leakage," flatulence, and abdominal cramping. Olestra was also shown to create a decrease in fat-soluble nutrients. [Neuhouser, et al. 2006]

Due to the fact that it caused so much digestive distress olestra rapidly lost its appeal as a fat substitute. While products no longer display its presence in bold letters on front-of-packaging labeling, it is still used in foods such as potato chips and "skinny" cookies. Read the label to avoid consuming this product.

Trans-fats, found in many fried fast foods and commercially prepared donuts, muffins, crackers, cookies, cakes, snacks, and artificial dairy products, have come under close scrutiny. Hydrogenation makes a liquid fat solid at room temperature. Once seen as a dietary darling, the addition of hydrogen to otherwise liquid unsaturated fats was actually believed to be better than saturated fats such as butter.

First created back in 1902, this hydrogenation process not only prevented the oil from spoiling, it extended the shelf life, making it a boon for manufacturers. In the 1950s it was presented as a way to reduce heart disease. (Remember the common assumption that margarine was healthier for you than butter?) In truth it turned out to be a dietary disaster: the Nurses' Health Study done by Harvard University showed that use of trans-fats actually increased heart disease. [Enig and Fallon. 2005] We now know that trans-fats not only lower HDL, or "good," cholesterol, but raises LDL, or "bad," cholesterol, a combination which is known to be bad for overall heart health. [Mayo Clinic. 2011]

Trans-fats became a mandatory part of the nutrition label in 2006 and dietary guidelines were set by the American Heart Association that limited intake to less than one percent of daily calories. In New York City Mayor Bloomberg passed regulations that limited the use of trans-fats in restaurants amid a huge outcry from restaurateurs. As it turns out these guidelines have had an effect, with one study showing a reduction in total cholesterol in children ages 6 to 19. [Kit, et al. 2012] According to an editorial published alongside the article, "A decrease in dietary trans-fats may be an important factor." [de Ferranti. 2012] It is important to remember, however, as mentioned in Chapter Two, governmental regulations allow manufacturers to claim that their products have zero grams of trans-fats if the amount per serving is less than .5. To avoid consumption of trans-fats you will need to read the label and make sure it does not contain the words "hydrogenated" or "partially hydrogenated," as these indicate trans-fats.

LABELING

When looking for healthy fats and cooking oils for your pantry the object is to aim for the best quality possible. As we'll discuss below this is not always a guarantee of a good product, but it is at least a place to start. If you are using butter, ghee, lard, or any of the animal fats you will want to read the label to ensure that these came from the best quality animal sources possible. Read about animal products in Chapter Seven to learn more about what you are looking for to determine the best quality.

There are a number of different terms that can be found on the label to describe oil quality and grade. These standards specifically apply to olive oil, and while they may be used for other oils there does not appear to be mandatory compliance.

DESCRIPTION	WHAT IT MEANS
Expeller pressed	A chemical free method of extracting the oils; no external heat is used.
Cold pressed	A chemical free method of extracting the oils; the environment is controlled and remains below 120ºF
Extra virgin	From the first pressing; unrefined
Virgin	Unrefined
Extra light	Often means refined; may be chemically treated to smooth out flavor and neutralize acidity
Pure	Often a blend of refined and virgin oils
Organic	From organic sources with no GMO product and no chemical pesticide or fertilizer

ADULTERATED OILS

In the wake of other food adulteration crises in China, the headline "Chinese Cooking Oil Found Contaminated" in March 2010 was simply the latest food safety scandal to come out of China. Drainage oil, made from refining kitchen waste, or oil with known carcinogens was found in as much as 10 percent of the cooking oil supply. [Greenhalgh. 2010] Two years later in January 2012 there was another investigation, this time for a producer who was mixing cottonseed oil and soybean oil with flavoring and selling it as peanut oil. [Reuters. 2012]

Any oil is potentially subject to adulteration and fraud. Olive oil has become one of the biggest food frauds due to its increasing popularity, high profitability, and the relative ease with which it can be adulterated. In fact, more olive oil is sold than is produced. Italy produces 400,000 tons of olive oil for domestic consumption, but 750,000 tons are sold. The difference is made up with highly refined nut and seed oils. Similarly, more oil is "produced" in California than there are olives available. The difference is made up with less expensive oils such as corn, soy, and sunflower.

Unfortunately this is one case where reading the label can't always help you make the best choice. According to a report of olive oils issued by the University of California, Davis, in July 2010, the majority of imported olive oils that were marked as "extra virgin" did not meet the standards, both domestically and internationally, for that label. Samples failed due to adulteration with cheaper oils, being made from poor quality olives, over-processing, and/or oxidization. While there were domestic oils that also failed, the percentage was not nearly as high. [Frankel, et al. 2010]

In the home environment there is no foolproof way to test for purity when it comes to olive oil. There is a theory that if you put some of the oil in a container in the refrigerator it will become more viscous or even semi-solid if it is pure, extra-virgin quality. Blended oils will not have the same response to refrigeration. This is, admittedly, not a very scientific way to test. A better option is to know and trust your source of olive oil. If you do not live in a state that produces olive oil, this may require purchasing online from a reputable company.

If you are concerned about possible adulteration of products it is important to stay well informed and to read the label to see where these products may be coming from. As of October 2012 Country of Origin Labeling rules were not mandatory for oils, however many are labeled. The challenge is to read the label and look beyond the "Product of…" label. There are situations where a product comes from somewhere else to be bottled in a more advantageous location. The label may also reveal the source of the ingredients that went into the oil. For example, an olive oil label may say, "Packed in Italy with select oils from Italy, Spain, and Tunisia." Do your research and learn which producers are creating product which is what the label claims it is or buy direct from a trusted producer.

SMOKE POINT

Different oils have different smoke points, when the oil begins to break down and produce smoke. While the smoke point can vary somewhat, depending on how refined and how pure the oil is, this generally limits what you can use an oil for. It is not recommended to use an oil above its smoke point as the breakdown of the oil can reduce the nutritional value. If you go too far above an oil's smoke point you can actually reach the flash point where it bursts into flames.

In the following table, I have listed various oils, including their smoke points and how to use them. This list does not include those I consider to be poor choices such as canola, corn, or soybean. For a basic oil suitable for cooking, sautéing, baking, and salad dressings, consider mixing together equal parts of extra virgin, cold pressed coconut oil and olive oil. This mixture should be shelf stable at room temperature.

OIL	SMOKE POINT	USES
Almond	430ºF	Baking, sautéing, stir frying, sauces, dressings
Avocado	520ºF	Frying, sautéing, dipping, dressings
Butter	302ºF	Cooking, baking, spread, sauces, dressings

OIL	SMOKE POINT	USES
Coconut	351°F	Baking, cooking, frying, spread, candy making
Flax Seed	225°F	Dressings
Ghee (clarified butter)	374-482°F	Deep frying, cooking, sautéing, condiment, dressing
Grapeseed	392°F	Sautéing, frying, dressings
Hazelnut	430°F	Dressing, sauces, baking
Hemp	329°F	Cooking, dressings
Lard	280-394°F	Baking, frying
Mustard	489°F	Cooking, frying, deep frying, dressings
Macadamia	410°F	Cooking, frying, deep frying, dressings
Olive, extra virgin	374°F	Cooking, sautéing, dressings, baking
Olive, virgin	419°F	Cooking, sautéing, dressings, baking
Palm	446°F	Cooking, sauces, dressings
Rice Bran	489°F	Cooking, frying, deep frying, dressings
Safflower	509°F	Cooking, dressings
Sesame	351°F	Cooking, dressings
Sunflower, high oleic	320°F	Cooking
Sunflower, linoleic	320°F	Cooking, dressings, baking
Walnut	399°F	Dressings, baking, sautéing

YOUR FAT ACTION PLAN

- Read the label to avoid fake fats (such as Olestra) and low-fat foods.

- Avoid soybean, canola, hydrogenated, and partially hydrogenated oils.

- Use oils for their intended purposes (do not go above the smoke point).

- Know your source to avoid adulterated oils.

CHAPTER SEVEN

Spending Wisely

"Organic food costs more! I can't afford it."

Often organic food does cost more, if you look only at the price on the product. Yes, an organic chicken costs more than that so-called "natural" chicken next to it in the meat case. But you also want to consider the value you are getting for your food dollars. How will your choice impact your health? After all, shouldn't that be our first concern when stocking our pantry? According to food journalist Michael Pollan, "The less we spend on food, the more we spend on health care."

This book is not intended to be a polemic for a pristine organic pantry. For most people it may not be practical or affordable to purchase 100 percent organic food. Often, choosing an organic product isn't necessary, unless you have a personal commitment to supporting the organic industry. Markets offer many fine and healthy alternatives that can help you balance your food budget.

Up to now, the chapters have looked at processed food choices and how to read the label to make an informed selection. In this chapter we will look to explore whole foods that are part of the pantry: such as our meats, dairy, eggs, vegetables, and more. Often these foods do not have the traditional nutrition labels, so there are new things to learn. Some of these definitions do apply to processed foods as well, although typically it is processed versions of the whole foods. I'll show you what the different options are in the various categories. While ultimately the decision to spend is yours, of course, the information presented in this chapter will help you make a more informed choice about your whole food purchasing options.

Conventional Foods are those foods raised according to standard agricultural practice. This usually indicates a use of pesticides and chemical fertilizers on the crops or on the feed that is given to animals. Conventional crops may also include GMOs, which are not labeled or identified in the US.

In November 2012 California voted on Proposition 37, a Mandatory Labeling of Genetically Engineered Food Initiative. In response to the ballot initiative many consumers got a good look at who owns some of the most popular organic brands, as Horizon, Silk, Kashi, Cascadian Farms, and others joined forces with Monsanto, DuPont, Dow Agriscience, and other biotech companies pouring financial resources into convincing voters to oppose Prop 37. Although these organic brands are prevented from using GMO foods in their products, their parent companies do use them in their other conventional brands (think Kellogg, Hershey, General Mills, Del Monte, J.M. Smucker, Ocean Spray, and others) and wanted to prevent consumers from knowing what's really in their food. They outspent the proponents of the labeling initiative by a factor of ten to one and Prop 37 was defeated. You can see an infographic highlighting this corporate ownership and the overwhelming amounts of money spent in this fight in Appendix Two. While the defeat of Prop 37 is a setback, it is certainly not the end of the issue.

In this country conventional agriculture also means animals in production for food can be given antibiotics, hormones, and other chemicals. Additionally conventionally raised animals are often raised in very tight quarters, which can promote illness or less than optimal development. Conventional standards are considered the norm, so meat products from conventionally raised animals are not labeled or identified. It is often the least expensive food option.

Natural is a difficult label to understand. There is an assumption that this label refers to foods that do not have any added chemicals or are not synthetic in any way. While there is an organization called the International Association of Natural Products Producers (IANPP) that is trying to create guidelines and definitions for this label, currently no standards are required. Because many people want minimally processed foods without added chemicals, but at a lower cost than organic, manufacturers frequently use this label. However, while there are a few—very few—regulations about using the natural label for meat products, there is absolutely no standard whatsoever for any other products using that label. According to the Cornucopia Institute, some manufacturers take advantage of the consumer's lack of knowledge by selling "natural" products, which are made with conventional ingredients at a price point similar to organic.

Organic is the description used for foods that are raised using a method of farming and gardening that relies on natural systems and products, and that avoids synthetic and toxic chemicals, fertilizers, and pesticides. There are comprehensive standards, called the Organic Production Act of 1990, for how products are grown, raised, and processed. The National Organic Program, a division of the USDA, oversees these standards. Foods that are raised according to organic methods cannot be genetically modified; cannot use pesticides, hormones, or other chemicals; and there are stricter guidelines for pasture-raised animals. Because GMOs are not clearly labeled or identified in this country, those people who do not wish to consume GMOs choose to purchase organic foods, since the standard does not allow for this type of contamination.

The issue, however, can be somewhat complicated. Just as producers do not want consumers to know whether their food contains GMO products, they also prefer that consumers not be very well informed about the issue. In September 2012 a study published by Stanford University appeared to indicate that there was not much difference between organic and conventional produce. The study essentially pointed out that there was virtually no nutritional difference between the two, concluding, "The published literature lacks strong evidence that organic foods are significantly more nutritious than conventional foods. Consumption of organic foods may reduce exposures to pesticide residues and antibiotic-resistant bacteria." [Smith-Spangler, et al. 2012]

According to information published just a short time later by the Cornucopia Institute, this study was issued with quite a bit of spin to it. Delving in to the Stanford study, the Cornucopia Institute pointed out that people also choose to purchase organic in order to avoid genetically engineered toxins and to reduce their exposure to agrochemicals. The study showed as much as an 81 percent reduction in exposure levels in organic foods, making this a significant reason to consider purchasing organic. A deeper review revealed missing information about pesticide residues and use of potentially carcinogenic chemicals, as well as the failure to include a 2011 study that showed GMO toxins accumulating in the bloodstream (rather than being excreted as is claimed by the biotechnology industry), indicating flaws with the study and a presumed scientific bias. Upon further examination, Cornucopia noted, there are strong financial ties between the school's Freeman Spogli Institute, which provided support for the researchers, and big agribusiness and biotechnology companies such as Monsanto and Cargill. [Cornucopia. 2012]

Many consumers don't realize that the label "natural" can include the use of GMO foods. The issue is further blurred when consumers rely on producers and grocery stores to keep them informed. In October 2012 a group called "Organic Spies" produced a video highlighting GMOs at Whole Foods. [Cornucopia. 2012] The video showed that many of the employees at Whole Foods were completely unaware of the presence of GMOs in some foods in the store. Some were even shown stating that there were no GMO products in the store at all. This misinformation makes it even more difficult for the consumer to know what they are eating.

Understanding what's in your food and the science behind the studies is important. Remember, another reason people choose to purchase organic products is that they believe the use of chemical fertilizers and pesticides is bad for the soil. Organic farming methods do not allow this use, making purchasing organic one way to avoid exposure through food to these chemicals. Many people also choose to purchase organic foods as mounting evidence seems to indicate that it is better for the environment, increasing biodiversity of species and promoting greater farm complexity, all of which are desirable outcomes. [Bengtsson, et al. 2005] [Norton, et al. 2008]

Organic foodstuffs tend to be more expensive than conventionally grown food. Paraphrasing hunorist Dave Barry, manufacturers and grocery stores have learned that consumers will buy anything, even floor polish, if it is labeled organic. Many people are committed to the holistic benefits that organic farming offers, and they consider their purchases an investment, not only in their families' health, but in the farmer and the planet. However there are plenty of conventionally grown, less expensive products that are safe to eat. At my local grocery store organic bananas are twenty-one cents per pound more expensive than conventional. Yet bananas do not need to be purchased organically. The peel helps to protect against pesticide residue and bananas are not a genetically modified crop. Learn which foods are most likely to be contaminated by pesticides or GMO and purchase those organic. For the others, such as fruits with a thick peel, save your money and purchase conventionally grown instead.

Sustainable farming is another method of food production. There are no standards or legislation in place, however, so a closer relationship with the farmer — to know how s/he is growing your food — may be required. Generally, no chemicals, antibiotics, hormones, or GMOs are used in sustainable farming. Sustainable farms tend to be run on a smaller scale, and the animals tend to have more room and time outside to follow their natural instincts in a healthy and comfortable setting. There are increasing numbers of farmers who choose to use sustainable methods, considering it an ecological philosophy. They need not meet the demands of an overseeing body with challenging and expensive standards and regulations to claim their products are sustainable. Some have also stated that the financial burden of organic certification makes it difficult for them to choose that, but they follow many of the same practices. One of the most well known sustainable farmers in the US is Joel Salatin, who runs Polyface Farm in Swoope, Virginia. He semi-jokingly refers to himself as a grass farmer since everything he does ultimately winds up somehow evolving around the grass, from the way the animals are pastured, to his crop rotations, to his soil amendments, and more.

Sourcing sustainably raised foods may be a little more difficult. I often find that the best way to identify them is to get to know your farmer either through a Community Supported Agriculture (CSA) program, or via farmers' markets. Talk to the farmers; ask them if they use pesticides and other chemicals or how their animals are raised. Some farmers may even invite the public to come visit them and see for themselves how the farm is run. Prices for sustainably raised products vary widely depending on where you live and what the availability is. Try shopping at your local farmers' market; you may find that the prices are much more reasonable than you expected.

When it comes to choosing between sustainable or organic, with the exception of those foods that are most likely to be GMO, I almost always opt for sustainable. These sustainable products are invariably local, and I prefer to support my smaller local farmers. I also find that by getting products produced nearby I am getting them at the peak of freshness — and nutritional value. Even organic food, if it has to travel far, will suffer the effects of being in a truck for a long distance, not to mention the ecological impact of transportation. It may also have been picked early, impacting flavor, texture, and nutrition.

THE HEALTHIEST BANG FOR YOUR BUCK

Now that you understand the different terminology, you may already be thinking about the options available in your area. Your grocery budget may be a necessary part of the equation. It's important to consider where to make choices in how you spend your food dollars while trying to keep your pantry as healthy as possible. Below I share some information for you to think about as you learn to balance these expenditures. You may not be able to make all of the suggested changes at once. Read through this chapter carefully and choose which ones are most important to you. Begin there, and as you are able, add in other options, either through making connections with your local farmer or discovering new places to shop where certain selections may be more affordable.

DAIRY

Choose organic or know your farmer when buying dairy products to avoid milk from animals treated with antibiotics and given GM feed laden with pesticides. Conventionally raised cows are often given an artificial hormone called Recombinant Bovine Growth Hormone (rBGH) or Recombinant Bovine Somatotropin (rBST). This hormone was invented by Monsanto and put into use in 1994 with the intention of having cows produce more milk. The US is the only premier nation in the world where rBGH is used; the European Union, Canada, Australia, and New Zealand do not allow it.

Not only does this artificial hormone cause cows to give more milk, it increases the health risks to the cows by increasing rates of mastitis (which then require antibiotics to treat the cow), and it has been known to cause cystic ovaries and uterine dysfunction in cows. rBGH also may be a problem, as it can reduce the pregnancy rate for cows that get the injections. [Epstein. 2006] A cow that cannot get pregnant will not, in industry terms, be "freshened," and therefore will be unable to give milk. Dairy cows that cannot give milk are sent to slaughter, as they are no longer able to continue their function.

It is important to remember that whatever hormones, antibiotics, or chemicals the cow is given do not go away when the cow is milked. Those chemicals are passed through the milk to those who consume it in products such as cheese, yogurt, and sour cream. Another serious side effect of rBGH in our milk is that it increases something called IGF-1, or Insulin-like Growth Factor-1, which is a hormone that may cause cancer. [Dona and Arvanitoyannis. 2009] And — a potential risk for young girls — there is some evidence that increased milk consumption may be related to the decreasing age at which many are starting to reach puberty. [Wiley. 2011] Although the study did not clearly identify if the milk was from cows given rBGH or not, certainly any exposure to added hormones and chemicals for developing children should be limited or avoided.

While there are dairy producers that label their products as rBGH-free, a move that Monsanto fought vigorously, the lack of this hormone still does not indicate a lack of antibiotics nor pesticides or GMO-laden feed. The only way to avoid those chemicals in your dairy products is to either purchase organic or make an effort to get to know your farmer and purchase sustainable dairy products locally.

Here is another reason to consider purchasing organic milk: laboratory measurements have shown that both protein and iron concentrations are higher in organic milk than are found in conventional milk. Additionally when fermenting milk (the process used to make either yogurt or kefir) the organic milk was found to have higher levels of conjugated linolenic acid (CLA) a fatty acid that has anti-cancer properties. [Florence, et al. 2009] [Parodi. 1999]

EGGS

Shoppers are confronted with an overwhelming array of choices when buying eggs. "Natural." "Cage free." "Vegetarian-fed." "Organic." "Omega-3." You get the idea. Read the labels to understand what's really going on. Producers will proudly proclaim that their eggs are from vegetarian fed chickens. And yet, as I mentioned earlier, chickens are not vegetarians, preferring to eat worms and bugs. Eggs from chickens who are allowed to roam freely and eat a natural diet are healthier. Additionally, many people assume that brown eggs are better. However, the color of an eggshell, brown, white, blue, or green, is determined strictly by the breed of chicken and has no bearing whatsoever on the nutritional value of the egg. The best, most nutritious eggs come from pastured hens allowed to roam and lay their eggs outside, scratching in the dirt and eating insects. Pastured chickens produce eggs higher in B12, folic acid, and omega-3s. These eggs are also lower in fat and cholesterol. [Long and Alterman. 2007]

Unfortunately there is no standard available to certify if the chickens are truly outside roaming freely, so the best way to get this type of egg is through your local CSA or farmers' markets. Growing numbers of people are looking to avoid the grocery store altogether when it comes to sourcing their eggs. Chickens are fairly easy to raise, and with more and more communities allowing urban chickens, many people are choosing to either raise their own or to participate in egg co-ops.

The following table provides some information about the meaning behind the different labels you might find on an egg carton:

EGG LABEL	INFORMATION
Regular (no special label)	These hens are fed conventional diets. Often they are warehoused in very small cages and receive no fresh air or sunlight. Many chickens are de-beaked to prevent them from pecking each other in their tight quarters.
Vegetarian Fed	These hens are probably raised the same way as the regular label hens above. They are fed a diet without bugs.
Certified Organic	While the hens usually are not caged and are fed according to organic standards, they may not have access to the outdoors. They are fed a vegetarian diet and may be de-beaked.
Cage Free	The chickens are not caged but usually do not have access to the outdoors. They can engage in natural behaviors. De-beaking is permitted.
Free Range	The chickens are not in cages and have some access to the outdoors, although there is no oversight for how much. Chickens can engage in natural behaviors. De-beaking is permitted.
Natural	This is a meaningless label, as there is no certification or oversight for it. These chickens are typically raised the same as chickens producing eggs with regular labels.
Omega-3 Enriched	This has no bearing on the living conditions of the chickens. They are fed a diet higher in omega-3s, usually from flaxseed. These chickens may be raised the same as chickens producing regular-label type eggs.
Pastured	Typically only available direct from the farmer, this term is used to indicate that the chickens are allowed full access to roam in pastures. Pastured is not the same as Free Range.

MEAT

As with dairy, I believe that it is important to purchase organic or sustainable meat products whenever financially possible. The reasons are the same as for dairy. Conventionally raised meat animals (and I'm referring to the most common meat animals here: cows, pigs, chickens, and turkeys) are often fed genetically modified and pesticide-laden feed. The addition of antibiotics to their feed can cause them to grow faster and to eat less, thereby making them more profitable for the producer. [Moore. 2011] These animals are also given enormous amounts of antibiotics to combat illness engendered by the concentrated animal feeding operation (CAFO), also referred to as a confined feedlot operation (CFO), or high density close quarters in which the animals are raised. This antibiotic use is troubling. According to reports published in *Food Safety News* in February 2011, the FDA revealed that 80 percent of all antibiotics used in the US are used in the food animal industry. [Bottemiller. 2011] In June 2010 the FDA began to urge farmers to use less antibiotics due to fears that overuse of antibiotics in animals could be leading to antibiotic-resistant bacteria. [Washington Post. 2010] [Gilchrist, et al. 2006] In April 2012 the FDA finally began to implement a plan requiring farmers and other animal producers to stop using antibiotics for growth purposes. They will now require a prescription so that antibiotics will only be given in the case of illness or health problems. [FDA. 2012]

Of equal concern is the use of arsenic in poultry feed. Originally added as a means of controlling a parasitical infection called coccidiosis, arsenic also caused chickens to get fat faster, and it made their meat look pinker (which we tend to think means it's healthier). Arsenic exposure can cause a wide variety of illnesses from diabetes and cardiovascular disease to a number of cancers, especially skin cancer, lung cancer, and bladder cancer. [Food and Water Watch. 2010]

The problem is further compounded when the chicken by-products, the feather meal, bone meal, and manure, from these arsenic-fed chickens is used elsewhere. One example is the arsenic-laced poultry litter that is often used on rice fields as a fertilizer. The arsenic found in chicken manure easily converts to a water-soluble form, so when it is spread on rice paddies the rice takes it up very easily as it is released.

The Consumer's Union is lobbying the EPA, USDA, and the FDA to ban the use of arsenic in our food system. In the meantime you can follow their recommendations to reduce your exposure by rinsing your rice, cooking it in a six-to-one ratio and draining off the excess water before eating. [*Consumer Reports.* 2012]

Choosing meat that is not conventionally raised, while more expensive, is important to reducing your exposure to these startlingly high levels of antibiotics and chemicals in your food. As stated in the section about dairy, whatever the animal consumes will, in turn, be consumed by you.

SEAFOOD

Seafood delivers cardio-protective levels of omega-3 fatty acids that are so important for our health. Seafood also provides a good source of iodine, which is important for thyroid health. However, not all seafood is the same, the quality can vary greatly due to a number of factors.

According to the FDA the US appetite for seafood is so great that more than 80 percent is imported. [FDA. 2009] It is worrisome that less than 2 percent of all imports are inspected, potentially exposing the consumer to higher levels of mercury, PCBs, antibiotics, and other environmental contaminants. [Becker and Upton. 2006] Another concern is whether the fish is wild-caught or raised in a farmed environment. As with land animals raised in a confined environment, fish suffer the ill effects of overcrowding when they are "farmed." Some of the challenges to keeping them healthy in this environment require giving them more antibiotics, which in turn can lead to bacterial resistance. [Chelossi, et al. 2003] Farmed fish are also more prone to parasitic sea lice, a condition that increases mortality and may be transmissible to wild fish populations. [Krkošek. 2006] Other illnesses from farmed fish include bacterial kidney disease and bacterial gill disease. [Bostick, et al. 2005] I believe it is reasonable to avoid farmed fish, especially from imports, as I do not feel that these unhealthy animals represent a high quality food source.

According to the Food and Water Watch, there is a "dirty dozen" for fish that should be avoided. These fish are: Atlantic cod, Atlantic flatfish (also known as halibut, flounder, and sole), caviar, Chilean sea bass, eel, farmed salmon, imported basa or swai or tra (sometimes sold as catfish), imported farmed shrimp, imported king crab, orange roughy, shark, and tuna (except for Pacific albacore and Atlantic skipjack).

Instead of these dirty dozen fish, your healthiest options are wild-caught cold-water fish. These would include: salmon, tuna (Pacific albacore and Atlantic skipjack), sardines, herring, anchovies, rainbow trout, and perch. Most canned tuna sold in the US is Pacific albacore (sold as "chunk white") or skipjack ("chunk light"). When purchasing these fish, always ask to see the label or some sort of tag showing that the fish is wild-caught and, if possible, sustainably fished using methods such as hand-line, troll, jig, or spear gun rather than habitat-damaging methods such as scraping, dragging, or blast fishing (i.e., using bombs to catch the fish). It is even better, for those who live near coastal areas, if your fish is caught locally according to these principles. Consider downloading the Smart Seafood Guide from The Food and Water Watch's website, the url is available in Appendix Four.

VEGETABLES AND FRUIT

Vegetables and fruits, while whole foods, are something to think about when you shop. There is a potential for certain products to be genetically modified but unlabeled; we'll talk about that below. The other issue is pesticide contamination. Conventional farming methods allow for the use of chemicals, in the form of pesticides and fertilizers, on or near these foods. Some foods are more likely than others to soak up those chemicals along with the nutrients they need to grow. The Environmental Working Group has compiled a list defining which foods are most likely to be affected in this way. These foods are called the "Dirty Dozen." Because they are not labeled, the only way to avoid these dirty dozen fruits and vegetables is to purchase organic versions. Conversely, there are foods that are least likely to be affected by pesticides, such as most foods with a peel; these are called the "Clean Fifteen." Corn is often considered a Clean Fifteen food. However, given the potential for GMO contamination, it is best to purchase organic corn. It is generally considered acceptable to purchase those foods conventionally, so you can save dollars there. [EWG. 2010]

> **The Dirty Dozen** fruits and vegetables are: apples, bell peppers, domestic blueberries, celery, corn, cucumbers, grapes, lettuce, imported nectarines, peaches, potatoes, spinach, and strawberries. Buy organic or sustainable versions of these foods if possible.

> **The Clean Fifteen** fruits and vegetables are: asparagus, avocados, bananas, cabbage, cantaloupe, eggplant, grapefruit, kiwi, mangoes, mushrooms, onions, pineapples, sweet peas, sweet potatoes, and watermelon. Corn is often considered a Clean Fifteen food. However, given the potential for GMO contamination, it is best to purchase organic corn.

One other way to identify organic produce is by the label. Conventionally raised produce has a four-digit PLU code starting with the number "4". Organic produce comes with a five-digit PLU code beginning with the number "9." According to Jeffrey Smith, a leading consumer advocate and executive director of the Institute for Responsible Technology, there is a myth that a five-digit PLU code starting with a number "8" means that product is genetically modified. Because the use of those codes is optional, producers don't use it, as many consumers would then choose to avoid those products. [Smith. 2010] If you want to avoid GMO produce, it is better to learn which foods are impacted and simply shop accordingly at the grocery store. The chart on page 88 produced by Bauman College, based on the Environmental Working Group's Dirty Dozen, is a good start. It also helps to identify healthy dietary intake for different food categories.

When shopping for organic produce at the grocery store, you may notice that the organic produce items in the green grocer section are separated from their conventionally raised counterparts. Legislation requires this separation to assure that any water run-off from the misters of the conventionally raised produce does not reach the organic produce.

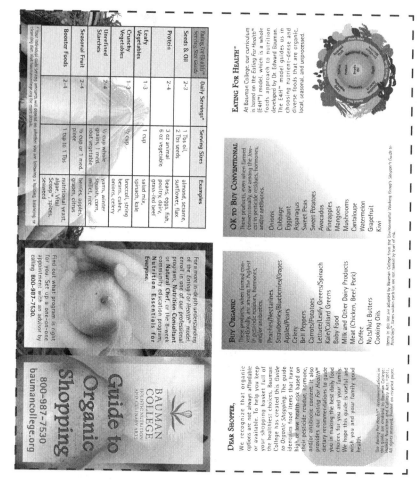

THIS GRAPHIC USED WITH PERMISSION OF BAUMAN COLLEGE

GENETICALLY MODIFIED ORGANISMS

Genetically modified organisms were initially created to make plants insect-resistant. Now foods are increasingly being genetically modified for many different reasons: to extend their shelf life, to make them resistant to viruses and to herbicides like Monsanto's Roundup, to create a weed-resistant plant, or even to add nutrients that do not naturally occur in that food, such as adding vitamin A to rice. Many scientists and others are concerned about the growing threat of cross-contamination by GMO crops. At least as early as 2001, examples were discovered of GMO contamination for unregulated, unapproved crops. [Halsberger. 2001] This is where GMO seeds spread to infect other fields or where crops cross-pollinate with non-GMO crops. This spread, this contamination, apparently cannot be contained.

Of equally serious concern is the increased potential for allergies from GMO foods due to proteins transferred from one food to another. One example of this was the discovery of a nut protein that appeared in GMO soybeans. [Nordlee, et al. 1996] For someone with a life-threatening allergy to nuts, this could be an extremely problematic issue. It is simple to stop eating nuts themselves but difficult to avoid them if you don't know where their proteins are hidden in your food.

According to the Institute for Responsible Technology the amount of GMOs present at the grocery store is overwhelming and continues to climb. The Institute for Responsible Technology currently estimates that 94 percent of all soy, 90 percent of all cotton, 90 percent of all canola, 95 percent of all sugar beets, more than 50 percent of Hawaiian papaya, and over 24,000 acres of zucchini and yellow squash are genetically modified. They also note the potential for GMO contamination in foods sources from animals that are given GMO feed. Even honey and bee pollen may be compromised if the bees have fed on GMO crops. Their Invisible GM Ingredients list inventories the vast number of probable genetically modified food products and additives. See Appendix Three for a complete list.

As I've mentioned before, there is nothing that requires a producer to tell you if their product is sourced from GMO items. The only way to avoid GMO at this point in time is to purchase organic. This is for all products made from these items. Due to the widespread "escape" of GMO canola in this country, many holistic practitioners go so far as to say that canola should be avoided altogether. [Schafer, et al. 2010]

Sadly, the spread of genetic modification of plants and animals continues to grow. New GMO foods that are currently seeking FDA approval include a salmon engineered to grow at twice the normal rate. [NYT. 2010] This is not a benefit to the consumer; it is a benefit to the producer who can raise more fish faster and make more profits. GMO alfalfa and sugar beets continue to be in the news. Both of these items were vigorously opposed; vast numbers of farmers objected to GMO alfalfa while a court order removed approval for GMO sugar beets.

Nevertheless, the USDA forged ahead and deregulated them. There are now no restrictions whatsoever on the production of genetically modified alfalfa. Of course, you probably don't eat alfalfa. But your meat and dairy products may have come from a cow that does. And a partial deregulation on sugar beets remains. [Grist. 2011] And in a bizarre move, one biotechnology company is seeking permission to produce a GMO apple that will not oxidize, or turn brown, when sliced. [ABCNews. 2010] The company fails to highlight the fact that the apple will also not turn brown when bruised, making it attractive and potentially more lucrative for vendors. I find this to be ludicrous, as a minimal amount of lemon juice will prevent oxidation for what I believe to be far less cost and with none of the dangers implicated in genetic manipulation.

Until such time as GMO labeling legislation becomes mandatory, the only way to avoid purchasing food containing GMOs is to buy organic, buy from a trusted source, grow your own from seed that you have verified is GMO-free, or to utilize the Non-GMO Shopping Guide. This guide is available free of charge online. See Appendix Four for more information.

As a reminder, the most highly genetically modified crops that we currently need to be aware of (and there may be more in the future) are: alfalfa, canola, corn, cotton, papaya, potatoes, soy, sugar beets, and zucchini and yellow squash.

YOUR FOOD BUDGET ACTION PLAN

If financially possible:

- Be aware of possible chemical, antibiotic, or hormone ingredients in or on your food.
- Choose organic or sustainably raised dairy.
- Choose organic or sustainably raised meat.
- Choose ocean-caught, sustainably harvested, wild fish.
- To avoid the Dirty Dozen fruits and vegetables, choose organic or purchase sustainably grown local produce.
- Choose organic for those products most likely to be genetically modified.

CHAPTER EIGHT

The Packaging

In 2011, a research organization conducted an eight-day study of five families who reported using canned and packaged food as part of their daily diets. At the beginning and end of the eight days, the families ate their usual diets. Then, for three days in the middle of the study, the families ate food that was prepared for them according to specific guidelines. All of the participating families received the same food. The majority of the food was from fresh and organic fruits, vegetables, grains, and meats. None of it came from cans. The preparation was done without plastic utensils or non-stick cookware. Food and drinks were stored in glass containers with BPA-free lids, and the food did not touch the lids. Even the coffee was made in ceramic or glass coffeemakers.

Urine samples showed that when the participants avoided plastic and ate primarily fresh foods, the levels of two toxic chemicals, BPA and DEHP, dropped by more than 50 percent in just three days. And when they resumed their normal diet, the participants' levels of toxins rose to levels measured at the beginning of the study. [Rudell, et al. 2011]

As this study showed, just as important as the ingredients added to the food are those that can be found in the packaging. Okay, so perhaps we can't all enlist the help of a personal chef to prepare and store our food like the participants in this study did. But plastic-free packaging is available to all.

These elements touch your food and can leach from the packaging into the food through various means (temperature, fat content, and time/exposure). Many of these substances are known to be obesogens, or endocrine-disrupting substances. Simply put, obesogens can cause weight gain by mimicking estrogen, unbalancing your hormones, and essentially reprogramming your metabolism. Additionally, when you consume obesogens it impacts your liver, which can lead to insulin resistance. This in turn causes your pancreas to pump out more insulin which puts further stress on your system and can, potentially, lead to diabetes. [Wang, et. al. 2011]

Below are a few of the most common packaging additives that can have a negative effect on your health, all of which should be reduced or eliminated from your pantry.

BHA AND BHT

Butylated Hydroxyanisole (BHA) is a petroleum-based preservative used as an antioxidant in many foods as well as a means of retarding rancidity in foods with oils or shortening. It can have a negative effect on the liver and the kidneys and, as far back as 1985, has been shown to cause cancer in rats. A 2011 Report on Carcinogens from the National Toxicology Program, Department of Health and Human Services, found BHA to be "reasonably anticipated to be a human carcinogen," however the FDA continues to label it as GRAS (Generally Regarded As Safe). Found in beverages, ice cream, candies, dry breakfast cereals, and more, BHA can also be found in packaging. Often appearing below the list of ingredients on the nutrition label, it may show up as a seemingly benign statement such as "BHA added to package for freshness." [Ito, et al. 1985] [NTP. 2011]

A related preservative, Butylated Hydroxytoluene (BHT) is also found in dry cereals as well as in chewing gum base and dry potato products. It is believed to be more toxic to the kidneys than BHA, having been shown to create kidney lesions in rats. BHT appears also to affect the brain, altering neurotransmitters. As far back as 1974 a study done at Loyola University revealed developmental changes to the offspring of mice who were fed BHT. These changes appeared to have an effect on the behavior of the offspring, which included negative impacts on sleeping habits, learning, and increased aggression. [Stokes and Scudder. 1974]

BPA

Bisphenol A is an endocrine-disrupting, estrogen-mimicking substance that has also been called obesogenic, meaning it can cause obesity. Studies show exposure to BPA can cause growth of breast cancer cells, increase the risk for heart disease, and is linked with obesity and other health concerns. [Qin, et al. 2012] [Melzer, et al. 2010] [Carwile and Michaels. 2011] A study of male factory workers appears to show a correlation between their exposure to BPA and impotence or erectile dysfunction while another study involving rats showed a reduction in serum testosterone after BPA exposure. [Ye, et al. 2011]

Its use in food-contact products such as can linings, baby bottles, and sippy cups has been questioned for a number of years. In 2010 in Canada it was declared to be a toxic substance, and the Canadian government began limiting its use. [Egan. 2010] In 2012 the FDA finally ruled that BPA could no longer be used in baby bottles or sippy cups but has, as yet, failed to limit its use in other applications such as can linings. [Tavernese. 2012]

BPA is insidious and can be found in a number of environmental sources. The biggest and most common source of BPA exposure is probably cash register receipts due to the thermal paper used to print them.

Even if you limit your canned goods to those with BPA-free linings or to foods packaged in glass, you still may have some exposure. The food may have been exposed elsewhere or the lid of the glass jar may be lined with BPA. Choosing containers that are less likely to have BPA is important to keep your levels as low as possible.

BPA-free plastics may not be a healthy alternative as recent studies appear to show that other bisphenols also have endocrine disrupting effects. [Viñas and Watson. 2013] Plastics, especially in food packaging, are so pervasive in our environment that it may not be possible to avoid them completely, however I believe it is important to limit your exposure as much as possible.

Folic acid can help negate BPA's effect on the body. Add foods rich in folate, such as beans and dark leafy greens to your diet.

Some companies are switching to alternative packaging, such as asceptic, or tetra pak cartons, for their products. Tetra paks are made with paper and low-density polyethylene (LDPE) a non-toxic plastic which appears to have no health impact. A few others have insisted their can suppliers and manufacturers make available BPA-free can linings for certain products.

Eden Foods is one company that packages their low-acid foods in BPA-free cans, and they are identified as such on the label. The company also uses glass jars for their high-acid crushed tomatoes and tomato sauces. Even the caps have a protective sealant. The company reports that this protective packaging increases the cost of their products, but that customers appreciate it and are willing to pay a little more for a safer package.

PERFLUOROCHEMICALS

Another family of man-made chemicals that appears in packaging is perfluorochemicals (PFCs). These are used to create products such as non-stick pans and oil-resistant food packaging (think microwave popcorn bags and fast-food burger wrappers). They also have non-food applications such as use in stain-resistant carpets, water-repellant fabrics, and the foam used to smother fires. There are a wide number of PFCs; perfluorooctane sulfonate, perfluorobutane sulfonate, and perfluorooctanoic acid (PFOA) are just a few. Essentially, anything starting with *perfluoro-* should be avoided.

The persistence of these chemicals in the environment and in our bodies is astounding, and one study showed that some have caused tumors and neonatal death and adversely affected the immune and endocrine systems in animals. Although the authors of the study were careful to point out that they believed the studies on the impact to humans brought only limited results, there were negative associations in people as well. And, as has been pointed out, we share a significant percentage of our DNA with mice, making it very reasonable to assume that what negatively affects them will also negatively affect us. [Steenland, et al. 2010]

One specific example deals with PFOA, which is used to make Teflon®, coat fast-food boxes, and line microwaveable bags. Teflon is available as a non-stick cookware; found on pots, pans, baking trays, and more, it is pervasive in stores and in homes across America. Consumers are often unaware of how much chemical contamination there can be with food that comes into contact with these substances. And the damage can be severe. It is startling to realize that in 2005, DuPont was fined $16.5 million dollars by the EPA after it was discovered that they hid approximately two decades worth of studies that revealed drinking water pollution, contamination of newborns, birth defects, and adverse effects to animals. In spite of the miniscule fine (at the time DuPont was worth approximately $25 billion dollars), this toxic substance is still being produced and is not due to be eliminated from the market until 2015. This represents a mind-boggling ten years after the contamination and pollution was discovered and approximately thirty years since this process began. [Eilperin. 2006]

ANTIMICROBIALS AND FUNGICIDES

Antimicrobial and fungicidal substances are used to extend the shelf life of food, killing and/or preventing the growth of pathogens, bacteria, and fungi in the food. Regulated by the FDA, there are definitions covering those substances that specifically come into contact with food. Some of the accepted food-contact antimicrobials are items we do not want in food, like sulfites and nitrates. However these substances can be made a part of the packaging and, according to a packaging industry source, "migrate into the food through diffusion." [Podhajny. 2001]

Antimicrobials are not marked on the label, making it difficult to know how much exposure you are getting. In order to limit their impact on your food and your health, it is best to repackage those foods that come wrapped in plastic films into glass or other safe containers. For raw meat products, if you are not going to use them within a day or two, it is best to freeze them until you are ready to cook them.

WHAT'S NEXT?

There are a number of new packaging options coming on to the market; more are likely to be developed over time. Many of these may not be marked on the label because packing is not a labeling requirement. The only way to know about these substances is to stay informed by using a source you trust.

SLIPS

Slippery Liquid Infused Porous Surface (SLIPS) is a new coating material created by scientists at Harvard University. An "omniphobic" material, it repels both water-based and oil-based materials. The purpose of this new coating is to ensure that all the food or liquid comes out of its container (although it appears to have other non-edible commercial uses such as potentially preventing airplane wings from icing over or pipes from accumulating sludge).

This technology may have marvelous potential for industry, and even for protecting your tablecloth from red-wine stains. But do we really want it coating the inside of a ketchup bottle? Yes, SLIPS may help you pour the last drops of ketchup onto your burger, but what toxins might come with it?

Based on a substance from a lotus plant, this new material is infused into a substrate, such as Teflon, and then used to coat the inside of containers. [Wong, et al. 2011] I do not know what the material is made from, whether it is a direct use of the plant material or, more likely, a chemical analog. Combined with the potential use of Teflon, this is another packaging material to be cautious of. Hopefully when SLIPS is commercially available, it will be clearly marked on the label, although given the lack of labeling for BPA this is doubtful. The only way to avoid this additive may be to pay attention to how well foods come out of their containers.

Seafood on Your Bananas

Packaging and coatings are a big deal when it comes to preventing food spoilage. An August 2012 article reported on the 244th National Meeting & Exposition of the American Chemical Society, where it was revealed that scientists have developed a new coating that, when sprayed on bananas, could delay the ripening process by up to two weeks. The product is made from chitosan, which is in turn made from shrimp and crab shells. In addition to making bananas unappealing to vegans and those who follow kosher dietary laws, this could present serious problems for those with high-level seafood allergies. Because seafood allergies are among the most dangerous ones, we can hope that this product will be labeled for those who need and/or choose to avoid it.

"Edible" Packaging

The newest packaging concept, still in development, encases a food in an edible skin. The bite-sized balls can hold a variety of otherwise-uncontainable foods, like yogurt, ice cream, and even juice and cocktails. Just rinse the ball as you would an apple or a carrot, and pop it in your mouth like a grape. The inventor claims the casing is biodegradable, with the raw ingredients coming from raspberries and algae. Of course algae tends to have free glutamic acid making a source of MSG. We also don't yet know what other ingredients make up the casing, so you don't necessarily want to eat them. These food balls are tentatively slated to appear in the US as early as 2013. You can be sure it will be accompanied by marketing spin. Be cautious of the hype; remember that biodegradable does not mean chemical-free. [Shapiro. 2012]

YOUR PACKAGING ACTION PLAN

- Read the label to see if additives have been noted in the packaging.
- When possible, choose additive-free packaging.
- Choose cookware that is not non-stick to avoid perfluorochemical coatings.
- Avoid prepared foods that come in coated packaging.
- Repackage foods in plastic coatings or coated containers once you bring them home.
- Eat more foods rich in folate to help against BPA exposure.

CHAPTER NINE

Pantry Makeover

R eading this book is a good way to understand many of the items that are in your pantry so you can choose what you no longer wish to use. But it's not always easy to visualize how to make those changes. As I've mentioned before, this book is meant to be a reference, something you can come back to over and over as you refine the contents of your pantry.

You might choose to use up the foods you already have, even if they are not the healthiest selections, and then replace them with more appropriate products. Or you might be inspired some Saturday morning to go through your kitchen and throw out everything that doesn't coincide with the *The Pantry Principle* guidelines.

Remember, following *The Pantry Principle* to create a healthy food source for your family is a step-by-step process, not an all-at-once endeavor. It takes time and effort to learn the necessary changes and to make substitutions. Start slowly. One night, read the labels on the food you prepare for dinner and make a note of those items you can purchase again and those you want to replace. On one shopping trip read the label on everything you put in your cart and compare it to the Seven Simple Rules list in Chapter One. Invite a friend over to go through your pantry and help you assess your stock. Then return the favor.

To help with this process I have put together a side-by-side comparison of a pantry from an actual client that reflects a typical American pantry and demonstrates *The Pantry Principle* makeover. Items are arranged alphabetically within a storage category, i.e., refrigerator, freezer, dry foods.

There are so many products available that, while I was able to use an actual pantry list and include brand names for this makeover, it is not possible to list all the varieties that would fall into the Pantry Principle. Instead, the Pantry Principle column identifies what you should look for as an alternative. The Notes column refers to reasons why you may not want to consume the products in the Typical Pantry column. I also have no particular brand loyalty and do not want you to simply follow the brand. Instead you need to rely on the skills you've learned. Read the label and understand the ingredients before you make your choice.

TYPICAL PANTRY	NOTES	PANTRY PRINCIPLE
REFRIGERATOR		
Apple juice drink, Snapple	Juice drinks are not juice Contains HFCS, most corn is GMO Contains Natural Flavors which could indicate MSG Apples are one of the most highly pesticide-laden fruits and vegetables	Choose 100% organic apple juice
Apples	Apples are one of the most highly pesticide-laden fruits and vegetables	Choose organic
Bell peppers	Bell peppers are one of the most highly pesticide-laden fruits and vegetables	Choose organic
Carrots	PP✓	PP✓
Celery	Celery is one of the most highly pesticide-laden fruits and vegetables	Choose organic
Cheese, Kraft sliced Swiss	Contains enzymes, which could indicate MSG Could contain artificial hormones Watch for the presence of artificial colors or annatto Cows may have been given GMO feed	Choose organic

TYPICAL PANTRY	NOTES	PANTRY PRINCIPLE
REFRIGERATOR		
Coffee Creamer, International Delights vanilla	Contains HFCS, most corn is GMO Contains flavor, two artificial sweeteners, artificial color, and a variety of chemical preservatives	Coconut milk and add your own vanilla
Cottage cheese, Breakstone	Could contain artificial hormones Contains Modified Food Starch and Natural Flavor, which may indicate the presence of MSG Cows may have been given GMO feed	Choose organic
Cream cheese, Philadelphia	Could contain artificial hormones Cows may have been given GMO feed	Choose organic
Cupcake icing, Betty Crocker, white	Contains trans-fats, artificial flavor, and sorbate Contains Modified Potato Starch, which may indicate the presence of MSG	Make at home
Deli sliced chicken	Many deli products contain nitrates; check the label	Choose nitrate free
Eggs	Refer to Chapter Seven, section on egg choices	
Homemade iced tea — plain	Remember to make healthy sweetener choices	PP✓

TYPICAL PANTRY	NOTES	PANTRY PRINCIPLE
REFRIGERATOR		
Homemade rhubarb jam	White sugar is often processed through bone char, not suitable for vegetarians or vegans Complex sugars do not affect blood sugar as quickly Look for cane sugar, as beet sugars may be GMO	Use a more complex sugar
Hot fudge, Smuckers	Contains HFCS, most corn is GMO Contains sorbates, and artificial flavor Contains Modified Cornstarch, which may indicate the presence of MSG	Make at home
Iceberg lettuce	Iceberg lettuce is nutritionally deficient	Choose romaine, green leaf, red leaf, Boston, or Bibb
Ketchup, Heinz	Contains HFCS, most corn is GMO	Choose HFCS-free ketchup
Lemonade, Minute Maid	Contains HFCS, most corn is GMO Contains benzoate, sorbate and artificial color Contains Natural Flavor and Modified Cornstarch, which may indicate the presence of MSG	Choose a different brand
Lemons and limes	**PP✓**	**PP✓**

TYPICAL PANTRY	NOTES	PANTRY PRINCIPLE
REFRIGERATOR		
Maraschino cherries	Contains HFCS, most corn is GMO Contains sorbate, benzoate, sulfur dioxide, and artificial color Contains Natural and Artificial Flavor, which may indicate MSG	Avoid
Miracle Whip	Contains HFCS, most corn is GMO Contains sorbate Contains Modified Food Starch, which may indicate MSG	Switch to mayonnaise with no unhealthy additives
Mustard, French's honey dijon	PP✓	PP✓
Olives, Kroger pimento stuffed	Contains alginate, chloride, and sorbate	Choose olives with no unhealthy additives
Organic miso	Be aware that miso contains free glutamates, the active ingredient in MSG	
Pears	PP✓	PP✓
Picante sauce, Pace	PP✓	PP✓
Pickles, Vlasic kosher baby dill	Contains Natural Flavor, which may indicate MSG Contains polysorbate 80, metabisulfate, chloride, and artificial color	Choose a different brand

TYPICAL PANTRY	NOTES	PANTRY PRINCIPLE
REFRIGERATOR		
Rice milk	Verify there is no carageenan	Choose unsweetened
Salsa, Pace chunky	Contains Natural Flavor, which may indicate MSG	Choose a different brand or make at home
Sour cream, Breakstone's	May contain artificial hormones Contains Natural Flavors and Enzymes, which may indicate MSG Cows may have been given GMO feed	Choose organic sour cream
Spaghetti sauce, Prego	Contains corn syrup and canola oil, both of which may be genetically modified	Choose a different brand or make at home
Tomatoes	Tomatoes do better when stored at room temperature rather than in the refrigerator	PP✓
Whole Milk, Hood	May contain artificial hormones Cow may have been given GMO feed	Choose organic
Wine	May contain sulfites	Choose sulfite-free wine
Yeast	Store in freezer for longer shelf life	PP✓

TYPICAL PANTRY	NOTES	PANTRY PRINCIPLE
REFRIGERATOR		
Yogurt, Yoplait flavored	Contains HFCS, most corn is GMO May contain artificial hormones Contains Modified Cornstarch, which may indicate MSG Contains annatto; allergic reaction possible Cows may have been given GMO feed	Choose plain, organic yogurt.
FREEZER		
Broccoli	PR✓	PR✓
Buckwheat flour	PR✓	PR✓
Burrito, Amy's Bean and Cheese	Contains annatto; allergic reaction possible	Look for colorant free choice
Butter	May contain artificial hormones	Choose organic butter
Chicken breasts, Tyson	Contains Yeast Extract and Modified Food Starch, which may indicate MSG Contains Polysorbate 80, caramel color, phosphate, and diacetate	Choose a different brand, preferably organic chicken
Corn	Most corn is GMO	Choose organic
Ice cream, Breyer's all natural cherry vanilla	May contain artificial hormones Cows may have been given GMO feed	Choose organic ice cream

TYPICAL PANTRY	NOTES	PANTRY PRINCIPLE
FREEZER		
Lasagna, Stouffer's	Contains bleached wheat flour Cheese may contain artificial hormones Contains Modified Cornstarch and Modified Food Starch, which may indicate MSG Most corn is GMO Cows may have been given GMO feed	Choose a different brand
Lemonade, Minute Maid	Contains HFCS, most corn is GMO Contains benzoate, sorbate and artificial color Contains Modified Cornstarch, which may indicate MSG	Choose a different brand
Lentil soup, homemade	PP✓	PP✓
Peas	PP✓	PP✓
Pizza, Stouffer's Lean Cuisine Three Meat	Contains enriched flour, nitrate, BHT, BHA, benzoate Cheese may contain artificial hormones Contains Modified Food Starch, which may indicate MSG Cows may have been given GMO feed	Choose a different brand
Pot Pie, Marie Calendar's creamy mushroom chicken	Contains trans-fats, MSG, dioxide, and caramel color	Choose a different brand

TYPICAL PANTRY	NOTES	PANTRY PRINCIPLE
FREEZER		
Sausage, Jimmy Dean	Contains MSG, artificial flavor, caramel color, and phosphate	Choose a different brand
DRY FOODS		
Applesauce, Mott's Cinnamon	Contains HFCS, most corn is GMO	Choose a different brand or make at home
Apricots, dried	Unless otherwise specifically stated, dried apricots contain sulfites	Choose sulfite free
Basmati rice, white	White rice has less fiber than brown rice; consider switching	**PP**✓
Black beans, Progresso	Contains Calcium Chloride May contain BPA	Choose a different brand or use dried beans
Cake mix, Betty Crocker	Contains enriched wheat flour, trans-fats, BHT, artificial flavor, artificial color, and chemical preservatives	Choose a different brand or make at home
Canola oil	Probably contaminated with GMO	Switch to olive oil or coconut oil
Cereal, Kashi Go Lean	Contains Textured Soy Protein which may indicate MSG Contains GMO ingredients	Choose a different brand

TYPICAL PANTRY	NOTES	PANTRY PRINCIPLE
DRY FOODS		
Cereal, Kellogg's Corn Flakes	Contains HFCS, most corn is GMO Contains BHT	Choose a different brand
Cereal, Special K	Contains HFCS, most corn is GMO Contains BHT	Choose a different brand
Cheese crackers, Goldfish	Contains artificial color Cheese may contain artificial hormones Cows may have been given GMO feed	Choose a different brand
Chicken broth, Swanson organic	Contains Autolyzed Yeast Extract, which indicates MSG Contains Natural Flavor, which may indicate MSG	Choose a different brand
Chicken in water, Hormel	Contains Modified Food Starch, which may indicate MSG Contains sodium phosphate May contain BPA	Choose a different brand
Cocoa powder, Hershey's	PP✓	PP✓
Coconut milk, Thai Kitchen	May contain BPA	
Coconut oil, Nutiva	May contain BPA	
Coconut shred, Baker's	Unless specifically stated, most dried coconut has sulfites	Choose unsweetened and unsulfured

TYPICAL PANTRY	NOTES	PANTRY PRINCIPLE
DRY FOODS		
Cooking wine, Holland	Contains sorbate and metabisulfate Very high in sodium	Use regular wine
Cornstarch	Most corn is GMO	Choose organic
Crystallized ginger	Use sparingly due to sugar content	PP✓
Curry spice mix, dry	PP✓	PP✓
Diced tomatoes, Hunts	May contain BPA	
Flour, unbleached all purpose, King Arthur	Use sparingly; choose whole wheat more often	Whole grains are a better source of fiber and better for health
Flour, whole wheat, King Arthur	PP✓	PP✓
Fruit Roll-ups	Contains corn syrup, trans-fats, monoglycerides, and artificial color Most corn is GMO	Choose a different brand
Granola bars, Nature Valley	Contains HFCS, most corn is GMO Contains Soy Protein Concentrate, indicating probable MSG	Choose a different brand or make at home
Honey	Heat processing destroys beneficial enzymes	Choose raw local honey

TYPICAL PANTRY	NOTES	PANTRY PRINCIPLE
DRY FOODS		
Italian Herb Seasoning	Contains trans fats Contains Whey Protein Concentrate, indicating probable MSG	Choose a different brand
Jam, Smuckers Simply Fruit strawberry	Contains Natural Flavors, which may indicate MSG	Choose a different product or make at home
Kidney beans, dry	PP✓	PP✓
Kidney beans, Eden organic	PP✓	PP✓
Lentils, dry	PP✓	PP✓
Noodles, Mother's	Whole grains are healthier than enriched wheat, durum wheat, or semolina pasta	Choose whole grain product
Nutritional Yeast, Red Star	Once open, store in the freezer	PP✓
Oatmeal Quaker Peaches and Cream Instant	Contains trans-fats, sulfites, and artificial flavor Whole grains are a better source of fiber and better for health	Choose Old Fashioned Oats for higher fiber content
Olive oil, Berio	PP✓	PP✓
Pasta, Barilla Multigrain	Multigrain does not mean whole grain Whole grains are a better source of fiber and better for health	Choose whole grain product

TYPICAL PANTRY	NOTES	PANTRY PRINCIPLE
DRY FOODS		
Peanut Butter, Skippy natural	Contains high amounts of sugar and oil May contain BPA	Choose a different brand Consider almond butter, which is a lower inflammatory food
Peaches, Libby's	May contain BPA	Always look for no added sugar
Popcorn	Most corn is GMO	Choose organic
Popcorn seasoning, Kernel Seasons	Contains Whey Protein Concentrate, Natural Flavor, Modified Food Starch, and Hydrolyzed Soy and Corn Protein probably indicating MSG Contains chemical preservatives	Use nutritional yeast
Pretzels, Goldfish	Contains Enriched Wheat Flour May contain canola or soy oils, both of which may be GMO	Choose a different brand
Quinoa	PP✓	PP✓
Raisins	Avoid golden raisins, which use sulfur dioxide	PP✓
Sesame seeds	Store in refrigerator for better shelf life	PP✓

TYPICAL PANTRY	NOTES	PANTRY PRINCIPLE
DRY FOODS		
Shitake Mushrooms, dry	**PR✓**	**PR✓**
Soup, Campbell's vegetable beef	Contains HFCS, most corn is GMO Contains MSG May contain BPA	Choose a different brand or make at home
Soup, Progresso vegetable	Contains MSG May contain BPA	Choose a different brand or make at home
Soy Sauce, Kikkoman	Contains MSG	
Sugar, white	White sugar is often processed through bone char, not suitable for vegetarians or vegans Complex sugars do not affect blood sugar as quickly Look for cane sugar, as beet sugars may be GMO	Choose more complex sugars
Tabasco	**PR✓**	**PR✓**
Tomato basil soup, Progresso	Contains corn syrup solids, most corn is GMO Contains bleached wheat flour Contains Modified Cornstarch May contain BPA	Choose a different brand
Tomato paste, Hunts	May contain BPA	

TYPICAL PANTRY	NOTES	PANTRY PRINCIPLE
DRY FOODS		
Tomatoes, Mezzetta sun dried	PP✓	PP✓
Tortilla Chips, Tostitos Natural	Most corn is GMO	Choose organic
Trail Mix, Chex	Contains Enriched Wheat Flour Contains trans-fats, artificial flavor, artificial color, and BHT	Choose a different brand
Tuna in water, Polar	May contain BPA	Look for wild caught
Vanilla, McCormick's	Be aware that some extracts contain caramel color and corn syrup, most corn is GMO	
Vinegar, apple cider, Eden	Choose raw and unfiltered	PP✓
Vinegar, red, Regina	Contains sulfur dioxide May contain sulfites	Choose a different brand
Vinegar, white, Regina	Contains sulfur dioxide May contain sulfites	Choose a different brand
Wakame (seaweed), Pacific	PP✓	PP✓
Walnuts, shelled	Store in the freezer for better shelf life	PP✓
Wasabi peas	Contains MSG and artificial color	Choose a different snack

TYPICAL PANTRY	NOTES	PANTRY PRINCIPLE
DRY FOODS		
Water chestnuts	May contain BPA	
Wheat Thins	Contains Enriched Wheat Flour Contains HFCS, most corn is GMO Contaims MSG, and artificial color Whole grains are a better source of fiber and better for health	Choose a different brand

Using the blank table on the following two pages create your own Pantry Principle Makeover list to help you remember the changes you want to make.

YOUR PANTRY	NOTES	PANTRY PRINCIPLE

YOUR PANTRY	NOTES	PANTRY PRINCIPLE

CHAPTER TEN

Taking The First Step

At this point you may have read the entire book and are feeling a little overwhelmed. You may be feeling like there is nothing you can eat without feeling guilty. You may be wondering if you can ever eat out again or go to eat at someone else's house. The answer is, yes you can.

As I have mentioned throughout the book, this is a step-by-step process. Figure out that one part of cleaning up your diet that is most important to you and start there. Everything you do, each change you make, is one thing more than you were doing before and something that will benefit your body. My story at the beginning of the book demonstrates how ill I was and how overwhelmed my body was. It took years of cleaning up my diet, one step at a time, to get to the point I am at today. And remember, I became a Nutrition Educator in the meantime!

If you throw out everything in your pantry and laboriously spend hours trying to re-fill your pantry, flipping through this book page by page, and then come home exhausted and overwhelmed after hours of shopping at the store, it will not be an exercise you will care to repeat. If instead you pick one thing that is important to you as a starting point, you will master that and learn how to remove those additives and other unwanted substances from your diet.

You want to strive for progress, not perfection. Don't get overwhelmed and discouraged. The point is that you are making mindful, well-considered decisions about your food and what you choose to eat. Give yourself time to integrate each change. Eventually it will become second nature to automatically choose brands that you know are healthy.

I encourage people to work on the principle of the 80/20 rule. If you can eat clean 80 percent of the time, with a few exceptions, your body can handle the rest. While it would be great to eat clean 100 percent of the time, it can be challenging to achieve.

The first step I strongly encourage people to take is to remove from their diets artificial colors (remember these are made from petrochemicals, a substance we do not need in our bodies), MSG (a potent neurotoxin), high fructose corn syrup, agave nectar, and artificial sweeteners. These are the ones I feel are most important to eliminate as completely as possible.

For the rest, the 80/20 rule is a reasonable expectation, it is achievable, and you can do it. It is important to remember orthorexia, which I mentioned in Chapter One, a condition involving high-level, overwhelming worry about your diet, which can lead to an unhealthy obsession with eating healthy food. That is not the purpose of this book. While it is important to be educated, informed, and aware, it is not healthy to be obsessive about your food.

Eating is not meant to be stressful or worrisome. It is one of our most pleasurable activities in life, either when shared or even when enjoying a simple, quiet, lovely meal alone. It is how we nourish ourselves, taking the time and the attention to care for our bodies. When we eat mindfully and slowly our bodies are fueled by the food, and we often find ourselves more satisfied by what we eat because we are paying attention. Being aware of our food, our bodies, and our mind is nourishment in itself.

There is a very powerful mind-body connection. When we rush through our meals we may find that we are startled by how quickly we ate. We may not even remember the taste or the sensations that go along with eating because we ate distractedly or in such a rushed fashion. When we eat slowly, mindfully, gratefully, we often find ourselves more satisfied with what we eat. Often we may find we need and want less food. [Hahn. 2011]

To recognize the mind-body connection, the next time you eat try the following exercise. After you have prepared your plate, set it in front of you on the table (not in front of the TV, the computer, or even a book) and look at it carefully. Look, really look, at the food on your plate. Appreciate the nourishment that is in front of you. With whatever utensil you are using to eat, bring it closer and notice if there is an aroma, some scent to the food. (Remember to take small bites, not huge mouthfuls.) Then put that first bite in your mouth. Hold it there for a second or two, appreciating the texture the food has in your mouth, noticing the rush of saliva, feeling the body reactions you may experience in reaction to the food in your mouth. S-l-o-w-l-y chew the food and notice how it tastes. Chew again, several more times, making the food into more of a thin paste before you swallow.

This mindfulness practice in eating offers several benefits. You will truly taste your food and enjoy it more. You will give your body time to recognize when it is full. You will appreciate the meal you spent time planning and preparing.

In addition to eating mindfully I encourage you to clean up your diet, one step at a time, picking whichever chapter is most important to you and working to implement the Pantry Principle. As you clean up your diet, as you make those changes, you will become comfortable with the changes you've made. When you've got that under control, when you feel you've mastered that section, move on to another one. Small, well-considered, meaningful modifications will turn into consistent, easily mastered changes.

CHAPTER ELEVEN

Recipes

You've read through this book and are engaged in reshaping your pantry to reflect the guidelines it offers. Now you are most likely looking at some of your choices and realizing that they no longer work for you. Along with that realization often comes the understanding that some of the food choices you were making, perhaps even the recipes you were using, rely far too heavily on over-processed, chemically laden packaged foods. As you begin to make changes in your pantry, you'll find yourself motivated to make changes to a number of your recipes.

Unfortunately, there is not nearly enough room in this book to share all of the wonderful and delicious new ways you can add whole foods to your diet. I do, however, have enough room to share a few favorites with you. I think you will find these dishes tasty, and they can give you some modest examples of how you can cast a more knowledgeable eye on some of your family favorites, re-creating them to be more in line with your new Pantry Principle.

As I've tried to caution—and comfort—you throughout this book, this is a journey, a step-by-step process. As you master the Pantry Principle, you will find yourself easily making changes to your recipes; one quite naturally leads to the other. Not only are you making different purchases, you have learned how to make substitutions and different choices in a number of ingredients. Some of those changes may happen several times as your recipes evolve along with your pantry. This is a good thing. You are creating healthy lifetime habits for you and your loved ones. If you have young children in your life, you are making powerful changes for their health and their future.

You and the other members of your family may also find a renewed sense of enjoyment in your food. As you clean up your pantry, so too you will clean up your palate, cleansing it of the overabundance of sugars often found in packaged foods and a distortion created by chemical contamination. These are things that can blunt our taste for food, causing us to become accustomed to them and unable to fully appreciate the abundance of taste and savor all that is whole food. I think you will agree this is an exciting change and, dare I say, a delicious benefit.

Let's eat!

RECIPE INDEX

BASIC PREPARATIONS

By learning how to make a few simple basics at home, you can avoid the processed versions at the store. Easy to do once you know how, these items when made at home will not have any of the added chemicals that you find in the grocery store versions. As an added benefit, the homemade versions are usually much less expensive.

Reconstituting Dry Beans

Canned beans often contain preservatives and come in BPA-lined cans. Reconstituting beans at home allows you to avoid these chemical additives. Dry beans swell to approximately three times their size. This means that two thirds of a cup of dried beans will reconstitute to two cups of cooked beans; the approximate amount found in a 15-ounce can. Although it does take longer, once beans are reconstituted they can be stored in containers in the freezer for up to six months and pulled out to use as needed. The whey in this recipe helps with digestibility. Note: do not add salt when reconstituting dry beans, as this will increase the cooking time and can cause the beans to be tough.

> **1 pound dry beans, any variety** (*this will make six cups of cooked beans*)
> **8 cups of water**
> **1 tablespoon liquid whey** (*See page 126 for how to make whey.*)

Sort the beans to remove any stones or other small debris. Rinse well to remove dirt and place into a large pot. Cover with water and bring to a boil. Cover pot and turn off heat. Let beans sit for two hours. Add whey and let beans sit 8 to10 more hours. Drain beans, rinse well, and return to the pot. Add clean water to the pot to cover the beans by 1 to 2 inches. Bring the beans to a boil. Reduce heat to low and simmer 60 to 90 minutes or until the beans are tender.

Bean Sprouts

You can make sprouts with just one type of bean, or make a mix. For mixes, using three to five different kinds works well. Bean sprouts are great in salads, stir fry, curry, smoothies (just a tiny bit for a protein boost). They also make a great raw snack.

5 tablespoons of dry beans
1 tablespoon liquid whey *(See page 126 for how to make whey.)*

Place beans into a colander and pick them over, discarding any small rocks, little clumps of dirt or other debris. Rinse the beans well. Place the beans into a bowl, add the whey, and cover them with water. Place the bowl in a draft-free place (the oven or microwave oven works well for this). Let them sit overnight. (If using your oven, be sure to put a note on it so you don't accidentally turn it on to pre-heat when your beans are in there. Trust me on this one.)

The next morning take your beans out of the oven and drain them. Rinse them well and put them back in the draft-free space overnight. The next day, rinse and drain your beans and put them back in the draft-free space. Repeat this process. On day two or three you will notice that your beans have little white sprout tails. On day three or four you will notice that lots of beans have sprouted, and they are ready to eat. How long they take to sprout depends on how warm or cold it is in your house. Once your sprouts are ready to eat, it's best to store them in the fridge.

Cooking Grains

When making rice it's a good idea to start by rinsing it first. This removes any loose starch and makes the end product much less sticky. If you are making sticky rice, it would still be rinsed, however you would use a specific variety called sweet rice or glutinous rice.

There is a concern about high levels of arsenic in rice. To reduce your exposure, consider cooking rice in a six-to-one ratio and draining off the excess water before eating.

Quinoa is a great option as an alternative to rice. It substitutes well in many of the dishes that call for rice (including the pilaf listed below) and has the added benefit of being a complete protein. When cooking quinoa it is important to read the label and see if it has been prewashed. Quinoa is coated in saponins, which can give it a soapy flavor if not washed off. If it has not been prewashed, you will need to soak your quinoa for 15 to 20 minutes before rinsing and cooking. You will also need a fine mesh strainer, as quinoa grains are very tiny.

Barley is a healthy, high-fiber grain with a delicious flavor and a chewy texture. Most barley in the grocery store is either quick-cook or pearled. Its hearty consistency works well in soups, side dishes, and stews.

COOKING METHOD

Measure and rinse your grain.

Using an appropriate size pot, add water and grain and bring it to a boil. Reduce heat to a simmer. Cover the pot with a lid cracked to allow steam to escape. When the pot is no longer steaming cover it fully. Let the pot sit the appropriate amount of time to cook

When the grain is done, remove the pot from the heat and let it sit 5 more minutes. Remove the grain from the pot to a serving dish and fluff with a fork before serving.

Do not leave the grain in the pot, as it can continue to cook from the residual heat.

GRAIN, 1 CUP	WATER	COOK TIME
Long grain, white rice	1 ½ cups	18 minutes
Long grain, brown rice	2 cups	50 minutes
Short grain, white rice	1 ½ cups	18 minutes
Short grain, brown rice	2 cups	50 minutes
Wild rice	2 cups	50 minutes
Red rice	2 cups	40 minutes
Black/Forbidden rice	2 cups	50 minutes
Quinoa	1 ¼ cups	35 minutes
Barley	2 cups	40 minutes

Quick Pilaf

A pilaf is a quick and easy way to make a side dish. By making a few simple changes to the cooking directions on the previous page, you can have a tasty addition to your meal.

use broth instead of water (*vegetable or chicken is fine*)
add 1 tablespoon of butter
add ½ teaspoon of salt
add 1 cup of diced vegetables (*suggestions include peas, mushrooms, celery, carrots, and/or green onions*)

Cook according to the chart listed above. When the pilaf is done mix in 1 tablespoon freshly minced parsley. Season with sea salt and fresh ground pepper to taste.

Polenta

Another grain-based food is polenta. It's so easy to make at home that you'll wonder why you ever bought it. The homemade version is much more versatile. By choosing organic cornmeal you can make GMO-free polenta.

1 cup cornmeal
1 teaspoon salt
3 cups water

Bring water and salt to a boil. Reduce water to a simmer and very slowly add cornmeal (*this is important to avoid lumps*). Cook approximately 20 minutes until mixture thickens. Remove from heat and pour into a pie plate (for triangles) or a cake pan (for squares).

Let polenta set for 10–15 minutes, cut and serve.

Chicken Soup Stock

Mineral-rich and very supportive to the body, this soup is a great way to use the chicken bones. The stock can be used as a starter for a meal, to cook rice or other grains, or as the basis of a soup. One delicious way to eat it is to simply warm up a cup and then season it with sea salt and freshly minced spring onions.

NOTE: This recipe can be doubled; however it may take longer to cook for the stock to reduce sufficiently to gel.

Bones from one organic chicken
Gizzards from an organic chicken
4 quarts of water
2 tablespoons of raw apple cider vinegar (*unfiltered and unpasteurized*)
1 large onion, quartered
3 carrots, cut into 1-inch pieces
4 ribs celery, cut into 1-inch pieces
5 cloves garlic, peeled
½ cup dry seaweed—*kombu, dulse, or kelp*
1 bunch parsley
1 teaspoon turmeric

Place chicken, gizzards, water, and vegetables except parsley into a large stockpot. Add vinegar and let the pot sit 30 to 45 minutes. Turn on the heat and bring mixture to a boil. Reduce heat to a simmer, cover, and cook 6 to 8 hours. Remove lid and skim foam from the top of the pot. Add the parsley and the turmeric. Cook another 30 minutes, uncovered.

Strain the stock into glass jars or containers. Refrigerate until stock is firm and fat has congealed. Skim fat from the top of the containers and discard.

Vegetable Soup Stock

For those who are vegetarian or who just want a vegetable soup, this is a wonderful way to create a rich-tasting broth. The potato peels and herbs add extra vitamin content, while the whey helps with digestion.

> 4 quarts of water
> 4 large organic potatoes, scrubbed and quartered
> 1 large onion, quartered
> 3 carrots, cut into 1-inch pieces
> 4 ribs celery, cut into 1-inch pieces
> 5 cloves garlic, peeled
> 2 bay leaves
> 1 bunch parsley
> 1 tablespoon thyme
> liquid whey (*See below for how to make whey.*)

Place all vegetables into a large stockpot and add water. Bring to a boil. Add herbs. Cover, reduce heat, and simmer 30–45 minutes. Blend all ingredients together to create a smooth consistency. Add 1 tablespoon of whey per cup of soup, stirring to blend completely.

Greek Style Yogurt (and Whey)

When straining yogurt to make the tangy, thick Greek style yogurt, the whey is separated out. This liquid can be used to soak beans and help reduce the phytic acids. It can also be used as part of the liquid in baking to help boost nutrition, or added to soups and smoothies.

> 1 32-ounce container organic whole milk yogurt

Line a colander with cheesecloth or an unbleached coffee filter. Place colander over a large bowl. Add yogurt. Loosely drape a kitchen towel over the top of the colander. Place colander and bowl in the refrigerator overnight. In the morning the colander will contain the thickened yogurt, while the bowl contains whey. Place each item into a separate container and store in the refrigerator. Refrigerated, the whey will last for up to six months, the yogurt will last until the expiration date on the original container.

CONDIMENTS

Many condiments contain a variety of undesirable ingredients, such as preservatives like potassium sorbate or calcium disodium EDTA. They can also frequently contain GMO ingredients, as the oils they tend to be made with are most often genetically modified: corn, canola, or soy. In the case of pesto, unless it's marked organic, the dairy product used may not be free of rBGH.

Fortunately, condiments are very easy to make, requiring just a few minutes to whip together. When made fresh, they often have a better flavor, making them a true compliment to the meal.

Mayonnaise

This recipe was inspired by my husband's grandmother, Mamie Lucienne. The end result is a delicious, creamy mayonnaise. It's a little thin at first, but after it sits in the refrigerator it firms up quite a bit and is just fabulous spread on sandwiches, in dressings, or any other way you choose to use mayo. This recipe should stay good for approximately two to three weeks in the refrigerator.

> 1 egg
> 1 cup olive oil, divided
> 1½ teaspoons dijon mustard
> 1 teaspoon sea salt
> 3 tablespoons tarragon vinegar *(can substitute white wine vinegar and a few fresh tarragon leaves)*

Place the egg, ¼ cup oil, mustard, and salt into a container. Blend well. *(A stick blender is the best tool for this.)* When well blended, drizzle in another ¼ cup olive oil and blend well again. Add the tarragon vinegar; blend well. Slowly add the remaining olive oil and blend well a final time.

Salsa

Salsa is rapidly becoming a favorite condiment for many people. Defined as a fresh relish, it's readily available on grocery store shelves. A very versatile sauce, it can be prepared in a variety of ways, with fruit, spicy, mild, any way you like.

More than just a dip for chips, salsa can be paired with many different foods:

- on top of baked potatoes
- mixed with brown rice and beans
- as a salad dressing
- on top of meatloaf
- with scrambled eggs in a taquito
- with baked chicken
- with baked fish
- use your imagination…the possibilities are endless

Starting with a basic salsa recipe, you can make changes however you like.

8 tomatoes, seeded and chopped
1 medium red onion, diced
1 red pepper, seeded and chopped
3–4 cloves garlic, minced
1 bunch cilantro, minced
½ teaspoon sea salt
½ teaspoon cumin powder
1 tablespoon lime juice

Mix all ingredients together and serve.

Pesto

Not just for pasta, pesto is a delicious way to add flavor to a wide number of dishes. It makes a fabulous sandwich spread, it's wonderful to use on chicken, and thinned down it is a great dressing for a cold bean salad.

Typically made with basil, pesto can be made to different flavor profiles by using other greens such as parsley, arugula, garlic scapes, or spinach. You can even substitute sun-dried tomatoes or roasted sweet bell peppers. Experiment and find out what your favorite flavor is.

2 cups fresh basil leaves, washed and de-stemmed
2 cloves garlic
½ cup organic Parmesan or pecorino Romano cheese
½ cup pine nuts or walnuts
½ cup olive oil
sea salt

Place all dry ingredients into a food processor. Turn the food processor on and begin to add in olive oil until mixture is smooth. Add salt to taste.

BEST EVER BREAKFAST

Serves 4

Polenta is a delicious, gluten-free dish made by cooking cornmeal in salted water. When making polenta, be sure to make enough for leftovers so you can enjoy this delicious breakfast. Just chill the leftovers in a lightly buttered bread pan and slice up the next morning. So simple and easy to put together, it's a fabulous and filling way to start your day. See Basic Preparations for cooking instructions.

> 3–4 tablespoons coconut oil, divided
> 4 slices polenta, ½-inch thick
> 8 ounces baby spinach, washed and drained
> 4 eggs
> 1 cup mushroom marinara
> nutritional yeast, sea salt, and fresh ground pepper to taste

In a large pan melt 1–2 tablespoons of coconut oil. When the oil is hot, add the polenta and fry 3–4 minutes until golden. Flip polenta and fry the other side. Place each polenta slice on an individual plate.

Add 1 tablespoon of coconut oil to the pan. Add baby spinach to the pan, tossing quickly, until it wilts. Divide spinach evenly and place on top of the polenta slices.

Add 1 tablespoon of coconut oil to the pan. Crack eggs and fry over easy *(cooked lightly, but not runny, on both sides)*. Place eggs on top of baby spinach.

Add mushroom marinara to the pan and heat through, approximately 1–2 minutes. Spoon mushroom marinara over the eggs. Top with a generous pinch of nutritional yeast. Add sea salt and pepper to taste.

BUCKWHEAT OAT PANCAKES

Makes approximately 10–12 five inch pancakes

Based on a recipe created by my friend Tina Berge, these pancakes are quick and easy to mix up. Denser and heartier than regular pancakes, they are a great high-fiber, filling way to start your morning.

When cooking pancakes or waffles, place the batches on a wire rack in your microwave oven while you cook the rest. The rack will keep the pancakes on the bottom from getting soggy, while the insulated space provided by the microwave oven helps to keep all of the pancakes warm.

½ cup buckwheat flour
⅓ cup oat flour
1 teaspoon baking powder
½ teaspoon baking soda
2 tablespoons ground flax seed
dash salt
2 large eggs
2 tablespoons melted coconut oil
1 tablespoon molasses
1 cup almond milk *(or enough to get desired consistency)*
blueberries or other add-ins, as desired

Mix flours, baking powder, baking soda, salt, and flax together in a medium bowl. In a small bowl, mix eggs, oil, molasses, and milk together. Gently mix egg mixture into flour mixture until thoroughly moistened. Let the batter sit for 10 minutes.

Pour pancakes into heated, oiled pan. Sprinkle with other toppings if desired. When pancakes show bubbles on the outside edge (not the whole top) flip and cook on the other side.

Crushed fruit, a thinned out jam, maple syrup, or honey are all delicious topping choices.

EVERYDAY BREAD

Makes 1 large loaf, or boule (a round loaf), or three small boules

This bread was created out of a desire to make a multi-grain bread that was easy and delicious. Soaking the grains helps to neutralize the phytates, which in turn makes the nutrients more available. This bread is slightly dense but still makes a great choice for everyday use in sandwiches, toast, and more.

NOTE: Kefir is a cultured milk product that is easily available in most grocery stores. If you do not have kefir, you can substitute either 1 cup of water with 1 tablespoon lemon juice or ⅔ cup of plain organic yogurt combined with ⅓ cup of water.

1 cup cornmeal
1 cup rolled oats
1 cup whole wheat flour
1 cup plain organic kefir
5 teaspoons of yeast
1 scant teaspoon ginger
1 cup warm water
1 tablespoon sea salt
2 tablespoons molasses
1½ cups all-purpose flour
olive oil for greasing dough

Mix together the first four ingredients and let rest 4–6 hours.

When ready to bake, mash together the yeast and ginger with the back of a spoon. Add water and mix well. Add the yeast mixture to the flour mixture. Add the sea salt and molasses and mix well, beginning to knead. Add the all-purpose flour a little at a time as required until dough is soft and no longer sticky. Knead dough for 8–10 minutes.

Oil the dough *(one method is to oil your hands and then rub them all over the dough)*. Place the dough in a bowl, cover with a clean dishtowel and let sit until double in bulk *(approximately one hour)*. Grease loaf pan or cookie sheet depending on if you are making a loaf or boules. Punch down dough and shape. Place into greased loaf pan or on greased cookie sheet. Let dough rise 30 minutes.

Place the pan into a cold oven. Heat oven to 400ºF. Bake the bread 35–45 minutes or until done. *(If you tap on the bottom of the loaf and it sounds hollow, it is done).*

Cool completely on a wire rack before slicing.

DIPS

Bean dips are a great snack. High in protein with a clean fat, they are quick and easy to make and so versatile. Often served with pita, crackers, or chips, these dips are great as a way to dress up a crudité plate. Served on endive leaves, in lettuce wraps, with celery, stuffed into cherry tomatoes, on cucumber slices, pepper slices, or with other vegetables, the choices are almost endless.

Hummus

2 cups cooked chickpeas
¼ cup water or whey
2–3 tablespoons lemon juice, depending on your preference
1½ tablespoons tahini
2 cloves garlic, crushed
½ teaspoon sea salt
2 tablespoons olive oil
paprika or fresh parsley for garnish

Combine chickpeas, water, and lemon juice/whey in a food processor. Blend together, slowly adding olive oil until the mixture starts to stick together. Add remaining ingredients and a little extra olive oil if needed to make it smooth.

Garnish with paprika or fresh parsley and serve.

Black Bean Dip

2 cups black beans
2 tablespoons raw apple cider vinegar
1 tablespoon lime juice
1 tablespoon olive oil
1 tablespoon chopped fresh cilantro
1 garlic clove, peeled
1 teaspoon ground cumin
sea salt and freshly ground pepper, to taste

Combine black beans, vinegar, and lime juice in a food processor. Blend together, slowly adding olive oil until the mixture starts to stick together. Add remaining ingredients and a little extra olive oil if needed to make it smooth.

Red Lentil Dip

This dip is a wonderful side to use warm with roast meats or vegetables. The lentils give it a bit of a protein boost, making it great for an afternoon snack. It's tasty when served cold with a collection of vegetable dippers such as endive leaves, zucchini slices, and slices of sweet bell pepper.

½ cup red lentils, rinsed and drained
1 cup water
1 medium carrot, sliced
1 small Vidalia sweet onion, sliced
2 cloves garlic, sliced
1 tablespoon chopped fresh parsley
1 tablespoon chopped fresh basil
1 tablespoon olive oil
½ teaspoon sea salt
pepper to taste

In a medium size pot, cook lentils in water. Bring to a boil and then reduce to a simmer. Simmer for 15 minutes, stirring frequently.

Remove from heat; it will look rather mushy. Set to cool for about 15 minutes.

Sauté carrots in the olive oil. Cook on medium until almost soft, approximately 10 minutes. Add onions and sauté another 2 minutes. Add garlic and sauté another minute. Add herbs and sauté another minute.

Put lentils, vegetables, and herbs in a food processor and blend until smooth. Season with salt and pepper. Delicious both warm and cold

Roasted Vegetable Dip

This dip is so delicious that, while we frequently eat it with sliced vegetables, we love it plain on crackers. My favorite is rice crackers with seaweed.

1 medium eggplant
1 yellow pepper
2 medium zucchini
1 medium Vidalia onion
2 teaspoons minced fresh thyme
2 teaspoons minced fresh rosemary
sea salt to taste
olive oil, as needed

Preheat the oven to 425°F.

Wash and slice vegetables into half-inch slices. Lay vegetable slices onto an ungreased cookie sheet. Drizzle lightly with extra virgin olive oil. Sprinkle with herbs *(but not salt)*. Roast in oven 35–40 minutes until vegetables are cooked and starting to brown. Place all vegetables into a blender or food processor and combine until smooth. Salt to taste. Transfer into a bowl and chill completely before serving.

GREAT GREEN SALAD

Serves 4

Adding more fresh food to your diet is important to good health, especially foods that have fiber, which supports good digestive function. This salad, with all of its juicy, crunchy components, provides a wide range of micronutrients as well as a delicious, healthy fat *(from the avocado)*.

1 Savoy cabbage, thinly sliced
½ English cucumber, diced
1 chayote squash, diced
2 ribs celery, diced
3 spring onions, white part only, diced
1 green apple, diced
1 avocado, cubed

In a large bowl, mix together all ingredients except avocado, blending well. Gently toss in avocado, being careful not to mash it too much while blending. Dress with lemon vinaigrette *(see following recipe)* and let sit a few minutes before serving

LEMON VINAIGRETTE

This bright-tasting vinaigrette is a wonderful addition to any salad. It can also be used over grilled fish or chicken as a tangy, tasty sauce.

NOTE: If you store leftover dressing in the refrigerator, be aware that the olive oil will congeal. The dressing will need to sit at room temperature before serving so that it will return to its liquid form.

¾ cup olive oil
¼ cup fresh squeezed lemon juice
½ teaspoon mustard powder
1 tablespoon minced fresh tarragon
½ teaspoon sea salt
a generous grating of fresh ground black pepper

Whisk lemon juice and seasonings together. Drizzle in olive oil while continuing to whisk to emulsify.

Alternate ways to emulsify dressing are to mix the ingredients using an immersion blender *(still drizzling in the olive oil)*, putting all the ingredients into a regular blender, or to put all of the ingredients together into a jar and shake vigorously until well combined.

CURRIED QUINOA SALAD

Serves 4

This is a great salad and goes well as a side at a barbeque. In our family we've been known to eat it as a meal as part of a composed plate with roasted vegetables and crudités. The dressing is delicious and goes well on other salads if you are looking for that slightly curried flavor.

Remember to rinse the quinoa before cooking to remove the saponins; otherwise it will taste soapy.

> 1 cup quinoa
> 2 cups water
> ¼ cup organic Thompson's raisins
> ⅓ cup hot water
> 1 red bell pepper, diced
> 3 scallions, diced
> ½ cup chickpeas
> ½ cup green peas, fresh or thawed
> 3 tablespoons minced fresh cilantro

Rinse quinoa. Bring water to a boil. Add quinoa, reduce heat, and simmer until all water is absorbed.

Place raisins into a bowl and cover with hot water, soak 5–7 minutes. Drain raisins.

Mix all ingredients together in a large bowl. Toss with dressing *(see page 138).*

DRESSING

    3 tablespoons fresh lemon juice
    2 teaspoons curry powder
    ½ teaspoon sea salt
    ¼ teaspoon pepper
    ½ cup olive oil

Combine lemon juice, curry powder, sea salt, and pepper in a jar. Cap tightly and shake vigorously to combine ingredients. Uncap jar, add olive oil, recap, and shake vigorously to combine.

Pour dressing over salad. Toss to combine thoroughly. Let sit at room temperature for 1–2 hours for flavors to meld.

QUINOA TABBOULEH

Serves 6–8

A Middle Eastern salad dish, most tabbouleh is made with couscous and mint. In this recipe the mint is exchanged for cilantro, which makes a delicious change and gives it a bit of a kick. Using quinoa instead of bulghur wheat makes the recipe gluten-free and provides a boost of fiber, B vitamins, calcium, and iron; quinoa also has balanced amino acids, which gives it a good protein profile.

    2 cups cooked quinoa
    1 cup finely minced cilantro
    ½ cup minced parsley
    1 clove garlic, minced
    1 teaspoon sea salt
    1 cup cherry tomatoes, halved
    1 red pepper, small dice
    3 scallions, mostly white part, minced
    3 tablespoon fresh lemon juice
    2 tablespoons olive oil
    ¼ cup pine nuts

Mix ingredients together, stirring well.
Top with fresh ground pepper.

GAZPACHO

Serves 4

My oldest daughter, Sasha, and I were rummaging through the fridge one day trying to figure out what to make for lunch and realized that we had all of the ingredients to make gazpacho. This is a perfect meal in the heat of the summer. Cooling and flavorful, it is easy to make and a wonderful way to get a huge serving of healthy veggies into your day.

Sasha prefers it extra chunky; I prefer a smaller dice. Gazpacho can also be lightly blended so all of the ingredients merge together to make a smoother-style soup. Any way you make it, it's delicious.

Dice and place in a large bowl:
1 large cucumber
2 large tomatoes
1 small Vidalia onion
1 sweet bell pepper
2 ribs celery
1 zucchini or yellow squash

Add in:
1 clove of garlic, crushed
¼ cup red wine vinegar
salt and pepper to taste

Cover with tomato juice. *(We didn't measure—just poured until it covered the veggies.)* Place in the refrigerator to chill for at least two hours.

To serve:
Ladle into a bowl. Drizzle with olive oil. Garnish with diced avocado and chopped cilantro.

LINCOLN POTATO SOUP

Serves 6

Quick and easy, this soup is a wonderful replacement for canned cream of potato soup without MSG, probable GMO corn, canola and soybean oils, or flavoring. The name for this soup came about when my daughter Veronica was little and misheard "leek and potato soup." My family has always loved this updated take on the classic. Adding cauliflower boosts the soup by including extra fiber, vitamin C, vitamin K, and folate.

> 3 tablespoons organic butter
> 1 bunch of leeks *(white part only)*, halved, cleaned, and chopped
>   *(note: there are usually 3–4 leeks in a bunch)*
> 1 large white or yellow onion, diced
> 4 cups organic vegetable broth
> 3 medium potatoes, peeled, rinsed and cut into
>   ½-inch thick slices
> 1 head cauliflower, broken up
> 1½ cups organic whole milk
> sea salt and pepper to taste

In a stockpot, melt the butter. Add the leeks and onions and sauté until they begin to soften. Add the broth, potatoes, and cauliflower to the pot and simmer, covered, 20 minutes or until tender. Using an immersion blender puree all the vegetables until smooth. Add milk, salt, and pepper.

This makes a fabulous meal when served with a salad and the Everyday Bread *(see page 132)*.

BREAD BOWLS

For an extra treat you can make a double batch of the Everyday Bread and bake six small boules.

After the boules are baked and cooled, preheat the oven to 350ºF.

Remove the top half-inch of the loaf. Remove most of the inner bread, leaving at least a one-inch lining, to form bowls. Baste the inside of the bowl with olive oil. Bake the bowls for 15 minutes. Remove from the oven and cool before filling. Serve the soup in the bowl.

The inside of the boule can be toasted and used for croutons or breadcrumbs.

MEATBALL SOUP

Serves 6

This delicious recipe came out of a combination of ingredients on hand in the fridge: chicken soup made from the bones of a roasted chicken, the outer leaves set aside from making fermented cabbage, the tops of celery, an onion, and the leftover bits of sweet bell pepper. It was a hit and is now a new family favorite.

> 1 medium onion, diced
> 1 clove garlic, minced
> 2 tablespoons olive oil
> 1 cup of diced celery *(mostly greens)*
> 8 large cabbage leaves, shredded
> ½ sweet bell pepper, diced
> 4 cups chicken broth
> 2 cups water
> meatballs *(see recipe below)*
> 1 cup cooked rice or quinoa
> sea salt and fresh ground pepper to taste

Heat olive oil in a large stock pot. Sauté onion until just starting to soften. Add garlic and sauté 1 minute. Add celery greens and shredded cabbage and sauté 2 minutes. Add bell pepper and sauté 1 minute. Add broth and water. Bring to just under boiling then reduce to a simmer. Gently spoon uncooked meatballs into the soup. Cook 20 minutes or until meatballs are done. Add rice, salt, and pepper and serve.

MEATBALLS

I use this recipe for a variety dishes—Swedish Meatballs, Hawaiian Meatballs, spaghetti sauce, and grinders; it's my go-to recipe. There are no breadcrumbs and we really don't miss them. The mixture comes out a little gloppy at first, but the meatballs are tender and juicy, which is just the way we like them.

This recipe doubles well. I usually double it so I can freeze some for later. My preferred mix is half ground turkey or chicken and half ground beef or bison.

> 1 pound organic ground meat
> 1 egg
> 1 tablespoon dried onion
> 1 tablespoon dried parsley
> ½ teaspoon dried oregano
> ½ teaspoon salt

Preheat oven to 350ºF. Mix ingredients together and form into golf ball sized meatballs. Bake for 20 minutes or until cooked through.

SLOW COOKER SPLIT PEA SOUP

Serves 6

The addition of the dulse, an edible seaweed found in the North Atlantic, to this recipe adds a wonderful flavor and a big boost of iodine and the other trace elements our bodies need. Making the soup in the slow cooker is a great way to have a hot meal ready to eat after a long day. When served with a salad and the Everyday Bread, this makes a very satisfying meal.

2 carrots, diced
2 ribs celery, diced
1 onion, diced
1 pound dried split peas, picked over and washed
2 tablespoons olive oil
1 bay leaf
1 tablespoon fresh thyme
6 cups water
1 teaspoon sea salt
¼ teaspoon fresh ground pepper
2 tablespoons dulse, crumbled

Place all ingredients except salt, pepper, and dulse in a slow cooker. Stir well to combine. Cover and cook on high for 6 hours. Remove bay leaf. Add salt and pepper. Blend together with an immersion blender. Ladle into bowls to serve and top with 1 teaspoon crumbled dulse.

CHICKEN CACCIATORE

Serves 4

Cacciatore means "hunter" in Italian. This braised dish was often made with either chicken or rabbit. Braising is a cooking method that combines both moist and dry heat. First the meat is seared over a high temperature, then left to cook slowly in liquid. Although typically made with bone-in meat and braised slowly for a longer period of time, this timesaver version uses boneless, skinless meat for a quick, satisfying dinner.

8 skinless, boneless, organic chicken thighs, rinsed and dried
2 tablespoons olive oil
sea salt and fresh ground pepper
½ teaspoon crushed red pepper flakes
3 cloves garlic, minced
1 yellow onion, diced
1 large bell pepper, diced
½ cup vegetable stock or red wine
1 28-ounce container crushed tomatoes
1 bay leaf
1 teaspoon minced fresh oregano
1 tablespoon capers, drained, optional
½ cup fresh parsley, chopped

In a large sauté pan, heat olive oil. Sear chicken 3–4 minutes on each side; remove from pan. Lightly dust chicken with salt and pepper, set aside. Add crushed red pepper and garlic to pan, sauté 1–2 minutes. Add onion and bell pepper and sauté 1–2 minutes until they start to soften. Add stock or wine, tomatoes, bay leaf, oregano, and chicken to the pan. Cook 5–10 minutes until chicken is done.

Remove from heat, add capers, if using, and let dish rest 5 minutes before serving.

Serve over polenta *(see recipe in Basic Preparations on page 124)* garnished with fresh parsley.

TUSCAN STEW

Serves 4

Lentils are tasty little legumes that pack a powerful nutrition punch. High in fiber, protein, folate, iron, potassium, and manganese, they are quick cooking and easy to use in a wide variety of dishes and cuisines. When combined with a grain such as rice, lentils provide a complete protein, as all of the essential amino acids are present.

This recipe is an Italian take on ratatouille, a French peasant stew, substituting the lentils for the eggplant to give a protein boost. Served over polenta *(see recipe in Basic Preparations on page 124)* with a side of spinach sautéed with garlic, lemon, and Italian spices it makes a fabulous meal. The leftovers, if there are any, are even better than the original, because the flavors continue to mellow and combine after cooking.

1 cup lentils, rinsed and picked over
1 onion, chopped small
3 cloves garlic, minced
3 zucchini, cut into half-inch slices
1 bell pepper, diced
3 tomatoes, diced
1½ teaspoons Italian herbs
½ teaspoon red pepper flakes
2 tablespoon olive oil
2½ cup vegetable stock

In a stockpot, heat olive oil and sauté onion and garlic until onion is starting to soften. Add the herbs and bell pepper and sauté 1 more minute. Add remaining ingredients and simmer on medium-low until lentils are done, about 30 minutes. You may need to add another one-half cup of stock. Salt to taste.

Serve over polenta and top with fresh grated parmesan cheese.

CRANBERRY OLIVE OIL BUNDT CAKE

Fresh cranberries offer a tasty tartness that is wonderful when cooked into homemade sauce or used in baking, such as in this fabulous Bundt cake.

Fresh cranberries can be frozen for use throughout the year. There is no need to wash or rinse them first; simply place into a freezer-safe container and freeze.

NOTE: You can also use blueberries instead of cranberries, simply omit the cinnamon and nutmeg.

6 egg whites
1½ cups evaporated cane juice crystals, a less refined suger
¾ cup extra virgin cold pressed olive oil
1 cup white whole wheat flour
1 cup all purpose flour
1 teaspoon baking soda
1 teaspoon salt
1 teaspoon ground cinnamon
½ teaspoon ground nutmeg
1 cup organic buttermilk
2 cups chopped fresh cranberries
2 tablespoons grated orange zest

Preheat oven to 350ºF.

Butter a 9-inch Bundt pan and dust with flour. In a bowl, beat the egg whites until stiff. Beat in the cane juice crystals until fluffy. Mix in the olive oil.

In a separate bowl, mix the flours, baking soda, salt, cinnamon, and nutmeg.

Alternately mix the egg white mixture and the buttermilk into the flour mixture until smooth. Fold in the cranberries and orange zest. Transfer the mixture to the prepared Bundt pan.

Bake 1 hour in the preheated oven, until a knife inserted in the cake comes out clean. Cook on a wire rack for 10 minutes. Remove from pan and top with glaze, below, if desired.

ORANGE JUICE GLAZE

1 cup evaporated cane juice crystals
¼ cup orange juice

Blend the cane juice crystals in a blender until finer and more powdery, Whisk together with orange juice and pour over the cake while still warm.

DIANA'S DELIGHTS

Makes approximately 30 cookies

These cookies were invented while playing in the kitchen with my youngest daughter, Diana. She loves chocolate chips and coconut. We wanted to create a cookie that was healthy, tasty, and easy to make. These have become a family favorite and are frequently the cookie of choice in our cookie jar.

½ cup organic butter
1 cup sucanat
1 egg
1 teaspoon pure vanilla extract
1 cup plus 2 tablespoons white whole wheat flour, sifted
½ teaspoon salt
½ teaspoon baking soda
1 cup rolled oats
½ cup semi-sweet chocolate chips
½ cup unsulfured, unsweetened shredded coconut

Preheat oven to 375°F. Grease cookie sheet.

Cream butter and sucanat together. Add egg, mixing well. Add flour, salt, and baking soda. Add oats, chocolate chips, and coconut.

Scoop teaspoon-sized balls of dough, roll into rounds, and place on greased cookie sheet. Bake 10 minutes in oven. Cool 2 minutes on cookie sheet before moving to wire rack.

TROPICAL TREASURES COOKIE

Makes approximately 30 cookies

I created this cookie for the book. I was so excited about reaching the funding goal necessary to help me self-publish that I went to play in the kitchen. Neighborhood kids were my taste testers and the response was overwhelmingly positive. I then held a naming contest and Annika Rockwell and Sara Faust were the winners.

NOTE: This dough is very sticky and somewhat shiny-looking when you have finished with it. But keep going because the results are a moist, chewy, delicious cookie.

1¾ cups sucanat
¼ cup melted organic coconut oil
2 eggs
1 cup shredded carrots
½ cup Thompson's organic raisins
⅓ cup unsulfured, unsweetened shredded coconut
¼ cup ground flax seed
1 teaspoon baking powder
½ teaspoon baking soda
½ teaspoon salt
2 cups rolled oats, pulsed in a blender or food processor to break into smaller pieces but not so fine as to make flour
3 cups flour

Preheat oven to 350°F. Grease cookie sheets with organic butter or coconut oil.

In a bowl combine sucanat and coconut oil. Stir until fully combined. Add eggs one at a time until fully combined. Add carrots, raisins, coconut, and flax; blend until fully combined. Add salt, baking soda, and baking powder; mix well. Add oats, blend until fully combined. Add flour; blend until fully combined.

Scoop teaspoon-sized balls of dough and drop on greased cookie sheet. Bake 10 minutes and remove from oven. Cool 4 minutes on cookie sheet before moving to wire rack.

APPENDICES

APPENDIX ONE

Sugars

Sugars can be found under a number of different names. One quick rule of thumb is that anything ending in -*ose* is usually a sugar; anything ending in -*ol* is typically a sugar alcohol. Beet or corn sugar and erythritol, unless they are organic, are probably GMO and should be avoided. Sugar alcohols do not have as many calories as sugar, however they do have calories and are therefore included on this list.

Because the list is so long it may be best to learn it a few names at a time, adding more as you are able.

ACCEPTABLE SUGARS	LESS DESIRABLE SUGARS
carob syrup	agave nectar
date sugar	barley malt
demerara	brown sugar
evaporated cane juice crystals	cane sugar
fruit juice	castor sugar
fruit juice concentrate	confectioner's sugar
honey	diastatic malt
jaggery	invert sugar
maple syrup	lactose
molasses	malt syrup
muscovado	palm sugar
papelon	rice syrup
piloncillo	sorghum syrup
rapadura	sucrose
stevia	sugar
tubinado	treacle
xylitol	

POTENTIALLY GMO SUGARS	SUGAR ALCOHOLS
beet sugar	arabitol
corn syrup	erythritol
corn syrup solids	ethyl maltol
crystalline fructose	glycerol
dextrose	isomalt
erythritol	lacitol
fructose	malitol
galactose	mannitol
glucose	sorbitol
glucose-fructose syrup	xylitol
high fructose corn syrup	
isoglucose	
maltodextrin	
maltose	

APPENDIX TWO

Who Owns Your Food?

The Cornucopia Institute is a non-profit organization that actively works to promote organic standards and regulations while also providing consumer education.

Cornucopia published the info-graphics on the following pages showing a clear chain of corporate ownership for many organic brands. The first info-graphic also identifies the money these corporations spent to prevent passage of Proposition 37, California's 2012 effort to require labeling of genetically modified food.

The chart on page 154 shows a clear chain of ownership by the top food producers. They want to own organic companies because consumers are demanding these foods, however as shown in the previous graphic, they don't want you to know what's in your food.

When we are at the grocery store it can be difficult to remember which company owns which. If you want to be able to avoid purchasing products from companies that helped to defeat Prop 37 the wallet card on page 155 from the Organic Consumers Association is a good place to start. Simply copy it, cut it out, and keep it in your wallet so it will be available when you are grocery shopping.

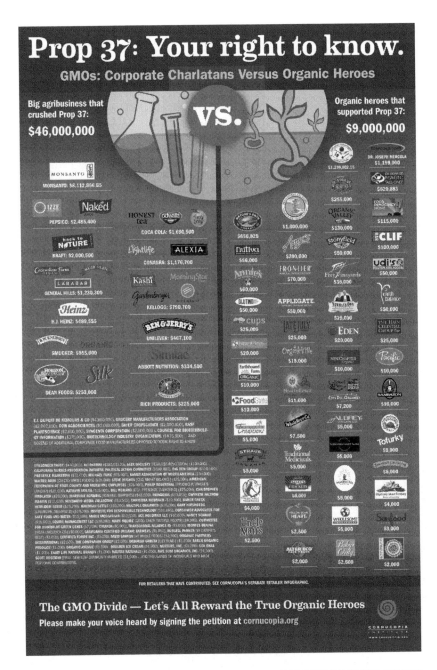

THIS GRAPHIC USED WITH PERMISSION OF THE CORNUCOPIA INSTITUTE

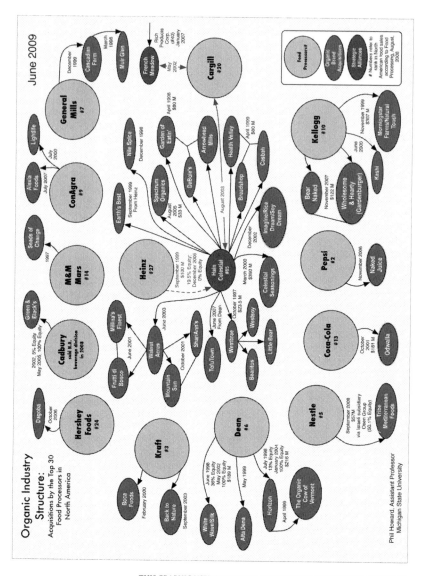

THIS GRAPHIC USED WITH PERMISSION OF THE CORNUCOPIA INSTITUTE

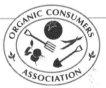
THIS GRAPHIC USED WITH PERMISSION OF THE ORGANIC CONSUMERS ASSOCIATION

APPENDIX THREE

Invisible GM Ingredients List

Aspartame
*(also called AminoSweet®,
NutraSweet®, Equal Spoonful®,
Canderel®, BeneVia®, E951)*

baking powder

canola oil *(rapeseed oil)*

caramel color

cellulose

citric acid

cobalamin (vitamin B12)

colorose

condensed milk

confectioners sugar

corn flour

corn masa

corn meal

corn oil

corn sugar

corn syrup

cornstarch

cottonseed oil

cyclodextrin

cystein

dextrin

dextrose

diacetyl

diglyceride

erythritol

Equal

food starch

fructose *(any form)*

glucose

glutamate

glutamic acid

glycerides

glycerin

glycerol

glycerol monooleate

glycine

hemicellulose

high fructose corn syrup (HFCS)

hydrogenated starch

hydrolyzed vegetable protein

inositol

inverse syrup

inversol

invert sugar

isoflavones

lactic acid

lecithin

leucine

lysine

malitol

malt

malt extract

malt syrup

maltodextrin

maltose

mannitol

methylcellulose

milk powder

milo starch

modified food starch

modified starch

mono and diglycerides

monosodium glutamate (MSG)

Nutrasweet

oleic acid

phenylalanine

phytic acid

protein isolate

shoyu

sorbitol

soy flour

soy isolates

soy lecithin

soy milk

soy oil

soy protein isolate

soy protein

soy sauce

starch

stearic acid

sugar
  (unless specified as cane sugar)

tamari

tempeh

teriyaki marinades

textured vegetable protein

threonine

tocopherols (vitamin E)

tofu

trehalose

triglyceride

vegetable fat

vegetable oil

vitamin B12

vitamin E

whey

whey powder

xanthan gum

Vitamin C (ascorbic acid), although usually derived from corn, is probably not GM because it is not likely made in North America.

TABLE USED WITH PERMISSION FROM THE INSTITUTE FOR RESPONSIBLE TECHNOLOGY

APPENDIX FOUR

Resources

The following is a list of organizations that provide information and/ or resources for consumers about whole foods, organic choices, environmental impact, and health matters.

Alliance for Natural Health USA
6931 Arlington Road, Suite 304
Bethesda, MD 20814
800.230.2762
http://www.anh-usa.org/

Center for Food Safety
660 Pennsylvania Ave, SE, #302
Washington, DC 20003
202.547.9359
http://www.centerforfoodsafety.org/

Center for Science in the Public Interest
1220 L St. N.W.
Suite 300
Washington, D.C. 20005
202.332.9110
http://www.cspinet.org

Cornucopia Institute
PO Box 126
Cornucopia, WI 54827
cultivate@cornucopia.org
608.625.2042
http://www.cornucopia.org

Environmental Working Group
1436 U Street. NW, Suite 100
Washington, DC 20009
202.667.6982
http://ewg.org

FarmMatch
http://www.farmmatch.com

Farm-to-Consumer Legal Defense Fund
8116 Arlington Blvd, Ste. 263
Falls Church, VA 22042
703.208.FARM (3276)
http://www.farmtoconsumer.org

Fed Up With Food Additives
http://fedup.com.au

Feingold Association
11849 Suncatcher Drive
Fishers, IN 46037
631.369.9340
http://feingold.org

Food and Water Watch
1616 P Street, NW Suite 300
Washington, DC 20036
202.683.2500
http://www.foodandwaterwatch.org

Holistic Moms Network
PO Box 408
Camden, NJ 07006
877.HOL.MOMS
http://www.holisticmoms.org/

Institute for Responsible Technology
PO Box 469
Fairfield, IA 52556
641.209.1765
http://www.responsibletechnology.org

International Organic Trade Resource Guide
28 Vernon St, Suite 413
Brattleboro, VT 05301
802.275.3800
http://globalorganictrade.org/index.php

Jamie Oliver's Food Revolution
http://www.jamieoliver.com/us/foundation/jamies-food-revolution/activists

Label Watch
http://LabelWatch.com

Local Harvest
http://www.localharvest.org/

MSG Truth
http://MSGTruth.org

Natural Resources Defense Council
40 West 20th Street
New York, NY 10011
212.727.2700
http://www.nrdc.org/

Non GMO Project
1200 Harris Avenue, Suite #305
Bellingham, WA 98225
877.358.9240
http://www.nongmoproject.org

Non GMO Shopping Guide
http://www.nongmoshoppingguide.com/

Organic Consumers Association
6771 South Silver Hill Drive
Finland, MN 55603
218.226.4164
http://www.organicconsumers.org

Pesticide Action Network, North America
1611 Telegraph Ave. Suite 1200
Oakland, CA 94612
510.788.9020
http://www.whatsonmyfood.com

Slow Food USA
68 Summit Street, 2B
Brooklyn, NY 11231
718.260.8000
http://slowfoodusa.org

Weston A. Price Foundation
5301 Dorsett Place Northwest
Washington, DC 20016
202.333.4325
http://westonaprice.org

BIBLIOGRAPHY

Abou-Donia MB, El-Masry EM, Abdel-Rahman AA, McLendon RE, and Schiffman SS. Splenda Alters Gut Microflora and Increases Intestinal P-Glycoprotein and Cytochrome P-450 in Male Rats. *Journal of Toxicology and Environmental Health*, Part A: Current Issues. Volume 71, Issue 21, 2008, Pages 1415 – 1429. doi:10.1080/15287390802328630.

Adulteration of Food. *The Cook's Guide and Housekeeper's & Butler's Assistant.* 2005. *http://www.thecooksguide.com/articles/adulteration.html*

American Botanical Council. *FDA Approves Stevia as a Safe Food.* Stevia.com. December 19, 2008. *http://www.stevia.com/stevia_article.aspx?/title=FDA_ Approves_Stevia_as_a_Safe_Food_Additive&id=8199*

American Chemical Society. Good news for banana lovers: Help may be on the way to slow that rapid over-ripening. *ScienceDaily.* August 22, 2012. *http://www.sciencedaily.com/releases/2012/08/120822100813.htm*

American Heart Association. *Sugar and Carbohydrates.* June 11, 2012. *http://www.heart.org/HEARTORG/GettingHealthy/NutritionCenter/ HealthyDietGoals/Sugars-and-Carbohydrates_UCM_303296_Article.jsp*

Assunção ML, Ferreira HS, dos Santos AF, Cabral CR Jr, Florêncio TM. Effects of dietary coconut oil on the biochemical and anthropometric profiles of women presenting abdominal obesity. *Lipids.* 2009 Jul;44(7):593-601. Epub 2009 May 13.

Baba T, Yoshida T, Yoshida T, and Cohen S. Suppression of Cell-Mediated Immune Reactions by Monosaccharides. *The Journal of Immunology.* March 1, 1979 vol. 122 no. 3 838-841.

Barnes, Brooks. Promoting Nutrition, Disney to Restrict Junk Food Ads. *NY Times.* June 5, 2012. *http://www.nytimes.com/2012/06/05/business/media/ in-nutrition-initiative-disney-to-restrict-advertising.html?pagewanted=all*

BBC News, Health. Artificial food colouring warning, May 8, 2007. *http:// news.bbc.co.uk/go/pr/fr/-/1/hi/health/6634071.stm*

BBC News World Edition. Fast food 'as addictive as heroin'. January 30, 2003. *http://news.bbc.co.uk/2/hi/health/2707143.stm*

Becker GS and Upton HF. Seafood Safety: Background and Issues. *Congressional Research Service Report for Congress*. April 3, 2009. *http://www.usvtc.org/trade/other/catfish/catfish.pdf*

Benard C, Cultrone A, Michel C, Rosales C, Segain JP, Lahaye M, Galmiche JP, Cherbut C, and Blottière HM. Degraded carrageenan causing colitis in rats induces TNF secretion and ICAM-1 upregulation in monocytes through NF-kappaB activation. PLOS ONE. 2010 Jan 13;5(1):e8666. PMCID: PMC2800179.

Bengtsson J, AHNSTRÖM J, Weibull A-C. The effects of organic agriculture on biodiversity and abundance: a meta-analysis. *Journal of Applied Ecology*. Volume 42, Issue 2, pages 261–269, April 2005. doi: 10.1111/j.1365-2664.2005.01005.x

Bigal ME and Krymchantowski AV. Migraine Triggered by Sucralose—A Case Report. *Headache: The Journal of Head and Face Pain*. Article first published online: 21 Mar 2006. doi: 10.1111/j.1526-4610.2006.00386_1.x

Blaylock, Russel L. Excitoxins: The Taste that Kills, Health Press. Santa Fe, NM. 1994. *Center for Science in the Public Interest*. FDA Urged to Prohibit Carcinogenic "Caramel Coloring". February 16, 2011. *http://www.cspinet.org/new/201102161.html*.

Bostick K, Clay J, and McNevin AA. Farm-level Issues in Aquaculture Certification: Salmon. *World Wildlife Fund FAO*. 2005. *http://tinyurl.com/bf8voyp*

Bottemiller, Helena. Most U.S. Antibiotics Go to Animal Agriculture. *Food Safety News*. February 24, 2011. *http://tinyurl.com/bgoufh2*

Brumfiel, Geoffrey. Genetically Modified Canola 'Escapes Farm Fields. *NPR*. August 6, 2010. *http://www.npr.org/templates/story/story.php?storyId=129010499*

Burdock, George A, Fenaroli's handbook of flavor ingredients. *CRC Press*. 2005. p. 277.

Cantazaro JM and Smith JG Jr. Propylene glycol dermatitis. *Journal of the American Academy of Dermatology*. Vol. 24, Issue 1, Pages 90-95. January 1991.

Carwile, Jenny L and Michels, Karin B. Urinary bisphenolA and obesity: NHANES 2003–2006. Environmental Research. Volume 111, Issue 6, August 2011. *http://tinyurl.com/c9k9vt5*

Center for Science in the Public Interest. Chemical Cuisine: Learn About Food Additives accessed January 8, 2010. *http://www.cspinet.com/reports/chemcuisine.htm*

Center for Science in the Public Interest. FDA Should Reconsider Aspartame Cancer Risk, Say Experts. June 25, 2007. *http://www.cspinet.org/new/200706251.html*

Center for Science in the Public Interest. Food Label Makeovers Proposed by CSPI. December 7, 2009. *http://www.cspinet.org/new/200912071.html*

Center for Science in the Public Interest. Parents Guide to Diet, ADHD and Behavior. 1999. *http://cspinet.org/new/adhd_bklt.pdf*

Chang JC, Wu MC, Liu I-M, and Cheng J-T. Increase of Insulin Sensitivity by Stevioside in Fructose-rich Chow-fed Rats. *Hormone and Metabolic Research.* 2005; 37(10):610-616. doi: 10.1055/s-2005-870528

Chelossi E, Vezzullib L, Milanoc A, Branzonic M, Fabianob M, Riccardia G, and Banat IM. Antibiotic resistance of benthic bacteria in fish-farm and control sediments of the Western Mediterranean. *Aquaculture.* Volume 219, Issues 1-4, 2 April 2003. doi:10.1016/S0044-8486(03)00016-4.

Choi H, Schmidbauer N, Spengler J, Bornehag C-G. Sources of Propylene Glycol and Glycol Ethers in Air at Home. *International Journal of Environmental Research and Public Health.* 2010. 7(12), 4213-4237. doi:10.3390/ijerph7124213.

Collison Kate S, Saleh Soad M, Bakheet Razan H, Al-Rabiah Rana K, Inglis Angela L, Makhoul Nadine J, Maqbool Zakia M, Zaidi Marya Zia, Al-Johi Mohammed A, and Al-Mohanna Futwan A. Diabetes of the Liver: The Link Between Nonalcoholic Fatty Liver Disease and HFCS-55. *Obesity.* Volume 17, Issue 11, pages 2003–2013, November 2009.

Consumer Reports. Arsenic in your food: our findings show a real need for federal standards for this toxin. Online ahead of print. November 2012. *http://www.consumerreports.org/cro/magazine/2012/11/arsenic-in-your-food/index.htm*

Cornucopia Institute. Food Grade Carageenan: Reviewing Potential Harmful Effects on Human Health; Executive Summary. 2012. *http://www.cornucopia.org/CornucopiaAnalysisofCarrageenanHealthImpacts042612.pdf*

Cornucopia Institute. NEW VIDEO: Organic Spies Goes Underground Looking at Whole Foods and GMOs. September 27th, 2012. *http://www.cornucopia.org/2012/09/new-video-organic-spies-goes-underground-looking-at-whole-foods-and-gmos/*

Cornucopia Institute. Stanford's Spin" on Organics Allegedly Tainted by Biotechnology Funding. September 12th, 2012. *http://www.cornucopia.org/2012/09/stanfords-spin-on-organics-allegedly-tainted-by-biotechnology 2-funding/*

Curezone. Food Additives — E–NUMBERS. nd. *http://curezone.com/foods/enumbers.asp*

Davidson T and Swithers S. Artificial sweetener may disrupt body's ability to count calories. *International Journal of Obesity,* 2004;28, 933–935. doi:10.1038/sj.ijo.0802660 Published online 27 April 2004.

de Ferranti, Sarah D. Declining Cholesterol Levels in US Youths. *Journal of the American Medical Association.* 2012;308(6):621-622. doi:10.1001/jama.2012.9621.

Di Justo, Patrick. What's Inside: For a Refreshing Hint of Tear Gas, Light Up a Cigarette. *Wired Magazine.* April 21, 2008.

Dininny, Shannon. USDA Asked to approve GMO Apple That Won't Turn Brown. *Bloomberg Businessweek.* November 29, 2010. *http://www.businessweek.com/ap/financialnews/D9JPLRR82.htm*

Dona A, and Arvanitoyannis IS. Health Risks of Genetically Modified Foods. *Critical Reviews in Food Science and Nutrition.* Volume 49, Issue 2, 2009, Pages 164 – 175.

Egan, Janet. Canada declares BPA toxic, sets stage for more bans. *Reuters.com.* October, 14, 2010. *http://www.reuters.com/article/2010/10/14/us-bpa-idUSTRE69D4MT20101014*

Eilperin, Juliet. Harmful Teflon Chemical To Be Eliminated by 2015. *The Washington Post.* January 26, 2006. *http://www.washingtonpost.com/wp-dyn/content/article/2006/01/25/AR2006012502041.html*

Emerald Performance Materials. Sodium Bezoate. *http://tinyurl.com/29w3yen*

Enig, Mary and Fallon, Sally. *Eat Fat, Lose Fat.* New York: Plume. 2005

Environmental Working Group. Shopping Guide. *http://www.foodnews.org/walletguide.php. 2010*

Epstein, Samuel S. *What's in Your Milk?: An Expose of Industry and Government Cover-Up on the Dangers of the Genetically Engineered (rBGH) Milk You're Drinking.* Bloomington, IN: Trafford Publishing. August 23, 2006.

Feingold Association of the United States. But aren't the FD&C dyes certified to be safe? nd. *http://feingold.org/certified.php*

Fife, Bruce. *The Coconut Oil Miracle*, Fourth Edition. New York: Avery. 2004.

Floch, M. Annatto, Diet, and The Irritable Bowel Syndrome. *Journal of Clinical Gastroenterology.* 2009 43:905-906. doi: 10.1097/MCG.0b013e3181b84517.

Florence ACR, da Silva RC, do Espirito Santa AP, Gioielli LA, Tamime AY, and de Oliveira MN. Increased CLA content in organic milk fermented by bifidobacteria or yoghurt cultures. *Dairy Science & Technology.* Volume 89 / No 6 (November-December 2009).

Food and Drug Administration. Guidance for Industry: Antimicrobial Food Additives. July 1999. *http://www.fda.gov/Food/GuidanceCompliance RegulatoryInformation/GuidanceDocuments/FoodIngredientsand Packaging/ucm077256.htm*

Food and Drug Administration. 2009 Approvals: Food and Color Additive Final Rules. Federal Register 74 FR 10483. Docket number FDA-1998-P-0032 (formerly 1998P-0724). 5/11/2010. *http://www.fda.gov/Food/FoodIngredientsPackaging/FoodAdditives/ucm074109.htm*

Food and Drug Administration. Chinese Seafood Imports. Don Kraemer Deputy Director Office of Food Safety, before U.S. and China Econimic and Security Review Commission. Last Updated 07/22/2009. *http://www.fda.gov/NewsEvents/Testimony/ucm115243.htm*

Food and Drug Administration. Code of Federal Regulations Title 21 Subchapter B – Food for Human Consumption Subpart G – Exemptions from Food Labeling Requirements. April 1, 2011. *http://www.accessdata.fda.gov/scripts/cdrh/cfdocs/cfcfr/CFRSearch.cfm?fr=101.100*

Food and Drug Administration. Color Additives: FDA's Regulatory Process and Historical Perspectives. Last Updated 12/17/2009. *http://www.fda.gov/ForIndustry/ColorAdditives/RegulatoryProcessHistoricalPerspectives/default.htm*

Food and Drug Administration. FDA Guide to Foods and Drugs with Sulfites. 2011. *http://extoxnet.orst.edu/faqs/additive/sulf_tbl.htm*

Food and Drug Administration. FDA takes steps to protect public health: Agency working with animal, drug and medical communities to promote judicious antimicrobial use. April 11, 2012. *http://www.fda.gov/NewsEvents/Newsroom/PressAnnouncements/ucm299802.htm*

Food and Drug Administration. Report on the Certification of Color Additives Foreign and Domestic Manufacturers. FYQ1 2000. Center for Food Safety and Applied Nutrition Office of Cosmetics and Colors. *http://www.fda.gov/ForIndustry/ColorAdditives/ColorCertification/ColorCertificationReports/ucm120693.htm*

Food and Drug Administration. Report on the Certification of Color Additives Foreign and Domestic Manufacturers. FYQ1 2011. Center for Food Safety and Applied Nutrition Office of Cosmetics and Colors. *http://www.fda.gov/ForIndustry/ColorAdditives/ColorCertification/ColorCertificationReports/ucm238762.htm*

Food and Drug Administration. Response to Petition from Corn Refiners Association to Authorize Corn Sugar as an Alternate Common or Usual Name for High Fructose Corn Syrup (HFCS), Letter to Mrs. Audrae Erickson, President, Corn Refiners Association. May 30, 2012. *http://www.fda.gov/AboutFDA/CentersOffices/OfficeofFoods/CFSAN/CFSANFOIAElectronicReadingRoom/ucm305226.htm*

Food and Water Watch. Milk Protein Concentrates. nd. *http://www.foodandwaterwatch.org/food/foodsafety/questionable-technologoies/milk-protein-concentrates/*

Food and Water Watch. Poison-Free Poultry: Why Arsenic Doesn't Belong In Chicken Feed. October 2010. *http://documents.foodandwaterwatch.org/doc/PoisonFreePoultry.pdf*

Food Intolerance Network. Food additives by code number | Colours. Last update April 2011. *http://fedup.com.au/images/stories/nastyadditive%20page.pdf*

Food Intolerance Network. Food Intolerance Network Factsheet – Annatto (160b). Updated September 2010. *http://fedup.com.au/factsheets/additive-and-natural-chemical-factsheets/160b-annatto*

Food Safety News. FDA Urged to Ban Cola Caramel Coloring. Feb 17, 2011. *http://tinyurl.com/axq6esv*

Fooducate. 1862-2011: A Brief History of Food and Nutrition Labeling. Updated February 2011. *http://www.fooducate.com/blog/2008/10/25/1862-2008-a-brief-history-of-food-and-nutrition-labeling/*

Frankel EN, Mailer RJ, Shoemaker CF, Wang SC, Flynn JD. Tests indicate that imported extra virgin" olive oil often fails international and USDA standards. *UC Davis Olive Center.* Robert Mondavi Institute for Wine and Food Science. University of California, Davis. July 2010.

Gilchrist MJ, Greko C, Wallinga DB, Beran GW, Riley DG, and Thorne PS. The Potential Role of Concentrated Animal Feeding Operations in Infectious Disease Epidemics and Antibiotic Resistance. *Environmental Health Perspectives.* 2007 February; 115(2): 313–316. doi: 10.1289/ehp.8837.

Great Vista Chemicals. Propyl Gallate. nd. *http://www.greatvistachemicals. com/industrial_and_specialty_chemicals/propyl_gallate.html*

Greenhalgh, Michelle. Chinese Cooking Oil Found Contaminated. *Food Safety News.* March 22, 2010. *http://www.foodsafetynews.com/2010/03/ contaminated-chinese-cooking-oil-supplies/*

Greig, JB. Who Food Additives Series 46:Cochineal Extract, Carmine, and Carminic Acid. *IPCS Inchem.* nd. *http://www.inchem.org/documents/jecfa/ jecmono/v46je03.htm*

Hahn, Thich Nhat and Cheung, Lillian. *Savor: Mindful Eating Mindful Life.* New York: HarperOne. 2011.

Haslberger, A. GMO contamination of seeds. *Nature Biotechnology.* July 1, 2001 19, 613. doi:10.1038/90201.

Henkel, J. From Shampoo to Cereal: Seeing to the Safety of Color Additives. *FDA Consumer.* U.S. Food and Drug Administration Center for Food Safety and Applied Nutrition. December 1993, Volume 27.

Hightower R, Baden C, Penzes E, Lund P, and Dunsmuir P. Expression of antifreeze proteins in transgenic plants. *Plant Molecular Biology.* 1991; Volume 17, Number 5,1013-1021. doi:10.1007/BF00037141.

Hord NG, Tang Y, and Bryan NS. Food sources of nitrates and nitrites: the physiologic context for potential health benefits. *American Journal of Clinical Nutrition.* 2009 Jul;90(1):1-10. Epub 2009 May 13. doi: 10.3945/ ajcn.2008.27131.

International Business Times. China makes fake rice from plastic. February 3, 2011. *http://www.ibtimes.com/articles/108582/20110203/china-makes-fake-rice-from-plastic-report.htm*

Ito N, Fukushima S, Tsuda H. Carcinogenicity and Modification of the Carcinogenic Response by bha, Bht, and Other Antioxidants. *Critical Reviews in Toxicology.* 1985;15:2, 109-150. doi:10.3109/10408448509029322.

Jaslow, Ryan. Colorado man Wayne Watson wins $7 million in popcorn lung lawsuit. *CBS News.* September 20, 2012. *http://tinyurl.com/92qmcn7*

Jaslow, Ryan. Starbucks Strawberry Frappuccinos dyed with crushed up cochineal bugs, report says. *CBS News.* March 27, 2012. *http://tinyurl.com/aw3n2tg*

Kit BK, Carroll MD, Lacher DA, Sorlie PD, DeJesus JM, Ogden CL. Trends in Serum Lipids Among US Youths Aged 6 to 19 Years, 1988-2010. *Journal of the American Medical Association.* 2012;308(6):591-600. doi:10.1001/jama.2012.9136.

Kobylewski, S and Jacobson, MF. Food Dyes A Rainbow of Risks. *Center for Science in the Public Interest.* June 2010.

Krkošek M, Lewis MA, Morton A, Frazer LN, and Volpe JP. Epizootics of wild fish induced by farm fish. *Proceedings of the National Academy of Sciences of the United States of America.* October 17, 2006 vol. 103no. 42. pnas.0603525103.

Lambert, Tim. A Brief History of Food. Last revised 2012. *http://www.localhistories.org/food.html*

Layton, Lyndsey. FDA seeks less use of antibiotics in animals to keep them effective for humans. *The Washington Post.* June 29, 2010. *http://www.washington post.com/wp-dyn/content/article/2010/06/28/AR2010062804973.html*

Lenoir M, Serre F, Cantin L, Ahmed SH. Intense Sweetness Surpasses Cocaine Reward. PLOS ONE. 2(8). 2007. e698. doi:10.1371/journal.pone.0000698.

Livestrong. Foods Containing Calcium Propionate. May 31, 2010. *http://www.livestrong.com/article/136250-foods-containing-calcium-propionate/*

Livestrong. Foods With Potassium Sorbate. 12/07/09. *http://www.livestrong.com/article/49380-foods-potassium-sorbate/*

Long, Cheryl and Alterman, Tabitha. Meet Real Free Range Eggs. *Mother Earth News*. October/November 2007. *http://www.motherearthnews.com/Real-Food/2007-10-01/Tests-Reveal-Healthier-Eggs.aspx*

Mann, Denise. Are Artificial Sweeteners Safe? *WebMD*. March 25, 2005. *http://www.webmd.com/food-recipes/features/are-artificial-sweeteners-safe*

Mayo clinic. Trans-fat is double trouble for your heart health. May 6, 2011. *http://www.mayoclinic.com/health/trans-fat/CL00032*.

McCann D, Barrett A, Cooper A, Crumpler D, Dalen L, Grimshaw K, Kitchin E, Lok K, Porteous L, Prince E, Sonuga-Barke E, Warner JO, and Stevenson J. Food additives and hyperactive behaviour in 3-year-old and 8/9-year-old children in the community: a randomised, double-blinded, placebo-controlled trial. *The Lancet*. Volume 370, Issue 9598, Pages 1560–1567, 3 November 2007. doi:10.1016/S0140-6736(07)61306-3.

Melzer D, Rice NE, Lewis C, Henley WE, Galloway TS. Association of Urinary Bisphenol A Concentration with Heart Disease: Evidence from NHANES 2003/06. PLOS ONE. January 2010; Volume 5, Issue 1.

Mercola, Joseph. This Sweetener Is Far Worse Than High Fructose Corn Syrup. *Huffington Post*. April 15, 2010. *http://www.huffingtonpost.com/dr-mercola/agave-this-sweetener-is-f_b_537936.html*

Mercola, Joseph and Kendra Degan Persall. *Sweet Deception: Why Splenda, NutraSweet, and the FDA May Be Hazardous to Your Health*. Corning, CA: Nelson Books. 2006.

Miller RR, Ayres JA, Calhoun LL, Young JT, and McKenna MJ. Comparative short-term inhalation toxicity of ethylene glycol monomethyl ether and propylene glycol monomethyl ether in rats and mice. *Toxicology and Applied Pharmacology*. Volume 61, Issue 3, December 1981. doi:10.1016/0041-008X (81)90358-6.

Moore, Michelle. Antibiotic resistant Staph bacteria found in meat. *Staph Infection Resources*. April 21, 2011. *http://www.staph-infection-resources.com/staph-mrsa-treatment/staph-bacteria-found-in-meat/*

More SS, Vartak AP, and Vince R. The Butter Flavorant, Diacetyl, Exacerbates β-Amyloid Cytotoxicity. *Chemical Research in Toxicology*. Publication Date (Web): June 25, 2012. doi:10.1021/tx3001016

Nakanishi Y, Tsuneyama K, Fujimoto M, Salunga TL, Nomoto K, An JL, Takano Y, Iizuka S, Nagata M, Suzuki W, Shimada T, Aburada M, Nakano M, Selmi C,Gershwin ME. Monosodium glutamate (MSG): a villain and promoter of liver inflammation and dysplasia. *J Autoimmun.* 2008 Feb-Mar;30(1-2):42-50. doi: 10.1016/j.jaut.2007.11.016.

National Toxicology Department. Report on Carcinogens, Twelfth Edition (2011); Butylated Hydroxyanisole. *Department of Health and Human Services.* 2011.

National Toxicology Program. NTP Toxicology and Carcinogenesis Studies of Polysorbate 80 (CAS No. 9005-65-6) in F344/N Rats and B6C3F1 Mice (Feed Studies). *National Toxicology Program.* Tech Rep Ser. 1992 Jan;415:1-225. PMID: 12616296.

Neuhouser ML, Rock CL, Kristal AR, Patterson RE, Neumark-Sztainer D, Cheskin LJ, and Thornquist MD. Olestra is associated with slight reductions in serum carotenoids but does not markedly influence serum fat-soluble vitamin concentrations1,24. *The American Journal of Clinical Nutrition.* March 2006 vol. 83 no. 3.

Neuman, William. Food Label Program to Suspend Operations. *New York Times.* October 23, 2009. *http://www.nytimes.com/2009/10/24/business/24food.html*

Newman, LC and Lipton, RB. Migraine MLT-Down: An Unusual Presentation of Migraine in Patients With Aspartame-Triggered Headaches. Headache: The Journal of Head and Face Pain. Volume 41, Issue 9, pages 899–901, October 2001. doi:10.1111/j.1526-4610.2001.01164.x.

Nordlee JA, Taylor SL, Townsend JA, Thomas LA, Bush RK. Identification of a Brazil-nut allergen in transgenic soybeans. *N Engl J Med.* 1996 Mar 14;334(11):688-92.

Norton L, Johnson P, Joys A, Stuart R, Chamberlain D, Feber R, Firbank L, Manley W, Wolfe M, Hart B, Mathews F, Macdonald D, and Fuller RJ. Consequences of organic and non-organic farming practices for field, farm and landscape complexity. *Agriculture, Ecosystems & Environment.* Volume 129, Issues 1–3, January 2009, Pages 221–227. doi:10.1016/j.agee.2008.09.002.

OSHA. Hazard Communication Guidance for Diacetyl and Food Flavorings Containing Diacetyl. *https://www.osha.gov/dsg/guidance/diacetyl-guidance.html.* 2012.

Paniagua JA, Gallego de la Sacristana A, Romero I, Vidal-Puig A, Latre JM, MD, Sanchez E, Perez-Martinez P, Lopez-Miranda J, and Perez-Jimenez F. Monounsaturated Fat–Rich Diet Prevents Central Body Fat Distribution and Decreases Postprandial Adiponectin Expression Induced by a Carbohydrate-Rich Diet in Insulin-Resistant Subjects. *Diabetes Care.* July 2007 vol. 30 no. 7 1717-1723.

Papazian, Ruth. Sulfites: Safe for Most, Dangerous for Some. *Ebsco Publishing.* April 2009. *https://igehrprodtim.med3000.com/PatientEd/html/13903.html*

Parodi, PW. Conjugated Linoleic Acid and Other Anticarcinogenic Agents of Bovine Milk Fat. *Journal of Dairy Science.* Volume 82, Issue 6, Pages 1339–1349, June 1999.

Philpott, Tom. USDA 'partially deregulates' GM sugar beets, defying court order. *Grist.* Feb 5, 2011. *http://www.grist.org/article/2011-02-05-usda-defies-court-order-partially-deregulates-gm-sugar-beets*

Podhajny, Richard M. Antimicrobial Additives and Coatings for Food Packaging. *Paper Film and Foil Converter. http://pffc-online.com/mag/1678-paper-antimicrobial-additives-coatings 2001*

Pollack, Andrew. Genetically Altered Salmon Get Closer to the Table. *New York Times.* June 25, 2010. *http://www.nytimes.com/2010/06/26/business/26salmon.html*

Pope Tara Parker. A New Name For High Fructose Corn Syrup. September 14, 2010. *http://well.blogs.nytimes.com/2010/09/14/a-new-name-for-high-fructose-corn-syrup/.*

Potera, Carol. Diet and Nutrition: The Artificial Food Dye Blues. *Environmental Health Perspectives.* 2010 October; 118(10): A428. pmcid: PMC2957945.

Public Citizen Health Research Group 1985. Dyes in Your Food. Edited by the *Feingold Association* in 2005. Published online 2011 March 30. doi: 10.1289/ehp.1003170. *http://www.feingold.org/Research/dyesinfood.html*

Qin XY, Fukuda T, Yang L, Zaha H, Akanuma H, Zeng Q, Yoshinaga J, and Sone H. Effects of bisphenol A exposure on the proliferation and senescence of normal human mammary epithelial cells. *Cancer Biology & Therapy.* Volume 13, Issue 5 March 2012. doi: 10.4161/cbt.18942.

R.J. Reynolds. R.J. Reynolds List of Ingredients (2010). *http://www.rjrt.com/TobaccoIngredients.aspx*

Reinberg, Steven. FDA Panel Delays Action on Dyes Used in Foods. *US News & World Report*. March 31, 2011. *http://tinyurl.com/abkp9eq*

Reuters. China seized 100 tons of melamine-laced milk powder. Aug. 21, 2010. *http://www.reuters.com/article/2010/08/21/us-china-health-milk-idUSTRE 67K0NO20100821*

Reuters. China probes another report of fake cooking oil. Jan 5, 2012. *http://www.reuters.com/article/2012/01/05/us-china-food-safety-idUSTRE 80416P20120105*

Rodrigues Florence AC, Claro da Silva R, do Espírito Santo AP, Gioielli LA, Tamime AY, and de Oliveira MN. Increased CLA content in organic milk fermented by bifidobacteria or yoghurt cultures. *Dairy Science Technology*. Volume 89, Number 6, November-December 2009. doi: 10.1051/dst/2009030.

Rudel RA, Gray JM, Engel CL, Rawsthorne TW, Dodson RE, Ackerman JM, Rizzo J, Nudelman JL, and Brody JG. Food Packaging and Bisphenol A and Bis(2-Ethylhexyl) Phthalate Exposure: Findings from a Dietary Intervention. *Environmental Health Perspectives*. 2011 July 1; 119(7): 914–920.

Schafer MG, Ross AX, Londo JP, Burdick CA, Lee EH, Travers, SE, Van de Water P, and Sagers CL. PS 103-166: Evidence for the establishment and persistence of genetically modified canola populations in the U.S. *Presented at the Global Warming ESA, 95th Annual Meeting*. August 6, 2010. Pittsburgh, PA.

ScienceDaily. Artificial Sweetener May Disrupt Body's Ability To Count Calories, According To New Study. June 30, 2004. *http://www.sciencedaily. com/releases/2004/06/040630081825.htm*

ScienceDaily. Too Much Fructose Could Leave Dieters Sugar Shocked. University of Florida. December 14, 2007. *http://www.sciencedaily.com/releases/ 2007/12/071212201311.htm*

ScienceDaily. Too Much Sugar Turns Off Gene That Controls Effects Of Sex Steroids. Child & Family Research Institute. November 21, 2007. *http://www. sciencedaily.com/releases/2007/11/071109171610.htm*

Shapiro, Ari Daniel. Packaging You Can Eat. *PRI's The World*. October 31, 2012. *http://www.theworld.org/2012/10/packaging-you-can-eat/*

Smith, Jeffrey. PLU Codes Do Not Indicate Genetically Modified Produce. *Huff Post Food*. 02/23/10. *http://www.huffingtonpost.com/jeffrey-smith/plu-codes-do-not-indicate_b_473088.html*

Smith-Spangler C, Brandeau ML, Hunter GE, Bavinger JC, Pearson M, Eschbach PJ; Sundaram V, Liu H, Schirmer P, Stave C, Olkin I, Bravata DM. Are Organic Foods Safer or Healthier Than Conventional Alternatives? *Annals of Internal Medicine.* 4 September 2012; volume 157 number 5.

Steenland K, Fletcher T, and Savitz DA. Epidemiologic Evidence on the Health Effects of Perfluorooctanoic Acid (PFOA). *Environmental Health Perspectives.* 118 (8) August 2010.

Stein, Herbert L. Annatto and IBS. *Journal of Clinical Gastroenterology.* 2009 43:1014-1015 Letters to the Editor. doi: 10.1097/MCG.0b013e3181ae4e1b

Stokes, John D. and Scudder, Charles L. The effect of butylated hydroxyanisole and butylated hydroxytoluene on behavioral development of mice. *Developmental Psychobiology.* 1974 Jul;7(4):343-50.

Strom, Stephanie. Walmart to Label Healthy Foods. *New York Times.* February 7, 2012. *http://www.nytimes.com/2012/02/08/business/walmart-to-add-great-for-you-label-to-healthy-foods.html*

Tannahill, Reay. *Food in History.* New York: Penguin Books. 1988

Tavernese, Sabrina. F.D.A. Makes It Official: BPA Can't Be Used in Baby Bottles and Cups. *New York Times.* July 17, 2012. *http://www.nytimes. com/2012/07/18/science/fda-bans-bpa-from-baby-bottles-and-sippy-cups. html?_r=0*

ToxNet — Toxicology Data Network. Citrus Red 2. 2003. 09/29/1994. *http:// toxnet.nlm.nih.gov/cgi-bin/sis/search/a?dbs+hsdb:@term+@DOCNO+2948.*

U.S. Census Bureau. Statistical Abstract of the United States: 2006. Table 202 Per Capita Consumption of Major Food Commodities: 1980 to 2003.

USDA. Chapter 2 Profiling Food Consumption in America. *Agriculture Fact Book 2001–2002.* nd. *http://www.usda.gov/factbook/chapter2.pdf*

United States Department of Labor. Occupational Safety & Health Administration. Hazard Communication Guidance For Diacetyl And Food Flavorings Containing Diacetyl. nd. *https://www.osha.gov/dsg/ guidance/diacetyl-guidance. html*

Viñas, R and Watson, CS. Bisphenol S Disrupts Estradiol-Induced Nongenomic Signaling in a Rat Pituitary Cell Line: Effects on Cell Functions. January 17, 2013. *Environmental Health Perspectives. http://ehp.niehs.nih. gov/2013/01/1205826/*

Walton, Marsha. Mice, men share 99 percent of genes. CNN. December 4, 2002. *http://edition.cnn.com/2002/TECH/science/12/04/coolsc.coolsc.mousegenome/.*

Wang T, Li M, Chen B, Xu M, Xu Y, Huang Y, Lu J, Chen Y, Wang W, Li X, Liu Y, Bi Y, Lai S, and Ning G. Urinary Bisphenol A (BPA) Concentration Associates with Obesity and Insulin Resistance. *Journal of Clinical Endocrinology & Metabolism.* February 1, 2012 vol. 97 no. 2E223-E227. *http://jcem.endojournals.org/content/97/2/E223.short*

Wansink, Brian. *Mindless Eating: Why We Eat More Than We Think.* New York: Bantam Books. 2006.

Washington Post. FDA seeks less use of antibiotics in animals. June 29, 2010. *http://www.washingtonpost.com/wp-dyn/content/article/2010/06/28/ AR2010062804973.htm.*

Wiley, Andrea S. Milk Intake and Total Dairy Consumption: Associations with Early Menarche in NHANES 1999-2004. *PLoS ONE.* February 14, 2011 6(2): e14685. doi:10.1371/journal.pone.0014685.

Winter, Ruth. *A Consumer's Dictionary of Food Additives, 7th Edition.* New York: Three Rivers Press. 2009.

Wong TS, Kang SH, Tang SK, Smythe EJ, Hatton BD, Grinthal A, and Aizenberg J. Bioinspired self-repairing slippery surfaces with pressure-stable omniphobicity. *Nature.* September 21, 2011. doi:10.1038/nature10447. 2011

Yang, Quin. Gain weight by going diet? Artificial sweeteners and the neurobiology of sugar cravings. *Yale Journal of Biology and Medicine.* 2010 June; 83(2): 101–108. pmcid: PMC2892765.

Ye L, Zhao B, Hu G, Chu Y, Ge RS. Inhibition of human and rat testicular steroidogenic enzyme activities by bisphenol A. *Toxicol Lett.* 2011 Nov 30;207(2):137-42. doi: 10.1016/j.toxlet.2011.09.001.

FUNDING PAGE

The generous support of the following people helped ensure that this book got published:

Lynne Aldrich

Kristen N. Bartolotta

Susan Blackmore

Vicki Bradley, Ph.D.

Mary Branson

Gloria A. Carr

Holly Caster

Lawrence Chalfin

Mary Chimarusti

Laura Connelly

Betsy and Drew Daubenspeck

Amy Day

Renee Devine

Sara Faust

Jodi Friedlander

Paul and Judy Glattstein

Seth and Kim Glattstein

Susan B. Glattstein

Joyce Greenlee

Tracy Greenwald

Cindi Hall

Betsy Healy

Krista Henkel-Selph

Joanne Herlihy

Sam and Jana Hopkins

Donna McGrath Householder

Dorothy Kennedy

Stephanie Knific

Maia Lagerstedt

Karen Langston, CNCP

Karen Levine

Charlie Lindahl

Shirley Locke

Bob Long

Larry and Stephanie Loomis-Price

Cyndie Mahaney

Michael Mangone

Mary Kay Masters

S. McBride

Heather McCrady

Terry Teague Meyer

Haya Meyerowitz

Hallie Moore

Donna Mosher

Jim and Linda Nadler

Carol Newman

S. Normand

Ben Orlove

Buffy Parker

Spiros Polemis

Helene Purdy

Thomas Quinlan

Padma Reddy

Sandra Reimold

Kate and Rusty Rhoad

Doris Richardson

Annika Rockwell, CN

Anita Smith

Trudy Scott, CN

Helen Sherwood

David and Priscilla Shontz

Lisa Singh

Sarah Smith

P. Snyder

Jennifer Strout

Ron and Limor Tager

Nancy Tague

Nikki Thai-Dessy

Peggy Walton

Claire Wang

There were a number of donors who did not wish to have their identities revealed publicly but who also contributed to this project.

To all of those who gave support, both listed and unlisted, I offer a heartfelt thank you.

INDEX

Made in the USA
San Bernardino, CA
20 April 2017